YOUNGER

YOUNGER

*The Breakthrough Anti-Aging Method
for Radiant Skin*

HAROLD LANCER, MD

FELLOW OF THE AMERICAN ACADEMY OF DERMATOLOGY

GRAND CENTRAL
Life & Style
NEW YORK • BOSTON

Grand Central Life & Style
Hachette Book Group
237 Park Avenue
New York, NY 10017

www.GrandCentralLifeandStyle.com

Printed in the United States of America

RRD-C

First Edition: February 2014
10 9 8 7 6 5 4 3 2 1

Grand Central Life & Style is an imprint of Grand Central Publishing.
The Grand Central Life & Style name and logo are trademarks of Hachette Book Group, Inc.

The Hachette Speakers Bureau provides a wide range of authors for speaking events. To find out more, go to www.HachetteSpeakersBureau.com or call (866) 376-6591.

The publisher is not responsible for websites (or their content) that are not owned by the publisher.

Library of Congress Cataloging-in-Publication Data

Lancer, Harold, author.

Younger : the breakthrough anti-aging method for radiant skin and total rejuvenation / Harold Lancer, MD, fellow of the American Academy of Dermatology ; with Diane Reverand.
     pages cm
Summary: "Renowned Beverly Hills dermatologist Dr. Harold Lancer is the expert on whom Hollywood's top celebrities rely to maintain their radiant complexions and to reverse the effects of aging. Now, he offers readers his groundbreaking, 3-Step Method to rejuvenate their skin at home. Based on years of clinical research, Dr. Lancer's regimen stimulates the skin's own transformative healing power for lasting results. He provides a road map to help readers navigate the mixed messages of today's dermatological advice, avoid expensive invasive treatments, and see through the empty promises of so many beauty products. He recommends the most effective skin care products for every budget from drugstores, department stores, and spas. He suggests surprising lifestyle choices in diet, exercise, and stress management that support beautiful skin. Whether the reader wants to maintain youthful skin or reverse the aging process, Dr. Lancer's Anti-Aging Method offers a comprehensive program for ageless, radiant skin."—Provided by publisher.
Includes bibliographical references and index.
ISBN 978-1-4555-4890-3 (hardback)—ISBN 978-1-4555-4892-7 (ebook)   1. Skin—Care and hygiene.   2. Beauty, Personal.   3. Health.   4. Nutrition.   I. Reverand, Diane, author.   II. Title.
RL87.L34 2014
646.7'2—dc23
                                                                              2013034406

To my tens of thousands of patients whom I have had the privilege of treating over the years and who have taught me so much in return.
Thank you.

Contents

Part Three

THE LANCER ANTI-AGING LIFESTYLE

Acknowledgments

First and foremost I must thank my family: my parents, Sara and Michael Lancer; my beloved wife, Dani; and my daughters, Alexis and Blair. Thank you for your unending love and support.

At Lancer Dermatology: A million thanks to my amazing, tireless staff and aestheticians, without whom I would be incapable of giving my many patients the individualized treatment they deserve—Nadia Aguilar, Natalie Aguilar, Susan Albovias, Beth Averion, Liliana Ayala, Mia Belle, Ruth Dela Cruz, Louise Deschamps, Yvonne Esformes, Vangie Equina, Michelle King, Melissa Medrano, Ram Prakash Khalsa (RPK), Tess Raymundo, Kat Rudu, and Marigil Santos.

At Lancer Skincare: Jeanne Chavez, Shannon Culhane, Jack Davies, Madeline Davis, Fanny DeCoster, Kenna Dworsky, and Alex Van De Leur, thank you for your tireless dedication to achieving my vision of the Lancer Skincare brand. To our wonderful publicists—Dara Busch, Jill Eisenstadt-Chayet, Jenny Halpern-Prince, and Richard Rubenstein—thank you.

To my *Younger* Team, Diana Baroni, Diane Reverand, David Vigliano, and the entire team at Grand Central Publishing, thank you for putting my professional vision down on paper. Ruba Abu-Nimah, Kevin Ley, Eric Nyquist, and Mary Schulte: Thank you for your creative contributions to *Younger*.

Ginger Bercaw, Carly Brien, Chris McMillan, Debi A. Monahan, Olivia Morgaine, and Gunnar Peterson, thank you for dedicating your time and for your expert contributions to the book.

Many thanks to Victoria Beckham, Simon Cowell, Ellen DeGeneres, Ryan Seacrest, and Oprah Winfrey for graciously disclosing that they enjoyed the care of my office and products, sending the Lancer line further than we ever thought possible.

A huge thank-you to Lisa Love, Tracy Margolies, Pat Saxby, and Peter Zimmerman for trusting the Lancer brand with their personal skin care and business.

Sarah Brown, Janelle Brown, Nicola Guarna, George Hammer, Vesa Kahlo, Cece King, Gemma Lionello, Marigay McKee, Anna Wintour, and Hazel Wyatt—thank you for your help in making the Lancer brand what it is today.

Finally, thank you to all of the professors at Brandeis University, UCSD Salk/Scripps Institute and School of Medicine, and Harvard University, as well as St. John's Hospital for Diseases of the Skin and Sheba Medical Center in Tel Aviv, for the invaluable knowledge, experience, and priceless education you endowed upon me.

A Note from the Author

Deep down, everyone wants to be beautiful. If you think about it, part of beauty is looking radiant and fresh, which is why just about everyone wants to look younger, too. The urge to be appealing transcends vanity. Attraction is the driving force in all of nature, a fundamental impulse in the physical world. We are hardwired to feel this way. It is in our DNA. The need to appear youthful and alluring is instinctive. Being desirable guarantees your survival, not to mention your contribution to future generations. Beauty elicits acceptance, admiration, and love from others. Being attractive heightens your power and influence. In other words, the world runs on the strong force of attraction or, as I like to call it, sex appeal. No wonder the annual global sales of beauty and personal care products have reached a staggering $426 billion and are rising, even with worldwide economic instability.

Soft, youthful skin, hair, and nails are the key components of physical beauty. Your skin is the first thing anyone and everyone notices. Luminous skin commands attention and outshines other qualities. A glowing, clear complexion at any age sends a message of health and vitality, the formula for attraction.

I have devoted the past thirty years to helping my patients make the most of their looks and erase years from their faces and bodies by dramatically improving their skin. I am a physician and surgeon with special training and certification in dermatology. I care for a roster of thirty thousand patients from around the world, an eclectic mix of all ethnicities from all walks of life. Since beginning my solo practice in 1983, I have treated all of my patients from beginning to end. Lancer Dermatology offers the most up-to-date medical, surgical, alternative, and cosmetic care at my Beverly Hills office, a wonderful space designed to be an oasis of comfort and beauty.

My philosophy of skin care is neither theoretical nor lab-based. Rather, direct experience in daily patient care for the past three decades has allowed me phenomenal opportunities for observation and creative solutions. My ideas and innovations have evolved from daily interaction with my patients. I have been dedicated to developing effective treatments for the many skin conditions that keep people from feeling and looking their best, and that includes the effects of aging.

I treat many A-list celebrities, whose privacy I respect. Even so, several stars have praised my skin care regimen and skin care products in the media. Oprah selected the Lancer Method Skincare products for her "2012 Favorite Things." The same year, Ellen DeGeneres included her personal favorites from Lancer Skincare in "Ellen's 12 Days of Giveaways."

The celebrities who come to me can choose anyone to care for their skin. I am honored that they put their famous faces in my hands and trust me to help them look their best. They are radiant, and their beauty remains their own. They know they will not leave my office looking as if they have spent a month in deep freeze or had a visit to the filling station. I take pride in knowing that my patients become the best version of themselves under my care with the invaluable help of the entire staff.

Experience is a great teacher. I have learned so much from being exposed to fifty to sixty patients a day. I see very few patients who are "dermatology virgins," who are consulting a dermatologist for the first time. My predecessors' evaluations help to mold my treatment strategies. After all, something was not working, which was why these patients came to consult with me. I now had the chance to solve their "derma-dilemmas," often complications resulting from invasive procedures. So many people today are looking for a quick fix and lose their judgment in the quest for eternal youth. The results are often disappointing, if not catastrophic. I see scars, bumps, crookedness, ripples, and countless other undesired outcomes. The cost is high, both figuratively and literally. Most of my new patients will never have a radical procedure again.

Twenty years ago, I had an epiphany that became the vision for how I practice dermatology today—my focus is on restoration, not alteration. I believe that the secret to beautiful skin has nothing to do with an artfully wielded laser, an injection, or cosmetic surgery. Lately, there has been so much focus on wrinkle freezers, line fillers, and lasers that no one considers what a simple high-quality skin care regimen can do for you. Glowing, healthy skin cannot be attributed solely to magic creams or even the gift of good genes. Genetic good fortune can take you only so far. The secret to an extraordinary complexion is your commitment to caring for your skin with my breakthrough three-step method—polish, cleanse, nourish—which I will reveal to you in this book. This program is the game changer that enhances the way your skin operates beneath the surface. The Lancer Method can improve the color, texture, elasticity, firmness, and hydration of your skin, and you do it at home in less than ten minutes a day.

In *Younger: The Breakthrough Anti-Aging Method for Radiant Skin*, I want to share the Lancer Method, which produces what is known in Beverly Hills as the Lancer Glow. As you will soon learn, the Lancer Method changes the focus of skin care. Skin care, as it is practiced by my colleagues and marketed by cosmetics companies, consists of quick fixes and false promises. Some people have never seen a blemish vanquisher, wrinkle reducer, skin plumper, eye circle eradicator, pore shrinker, redness reliever, line smoother, collagen builder, or super moisturizer that they did not want to try. Their bathroom drawers and cabinets are overflowing with their collection of expensive products. It is a scene from *Hoarders*. Nothing seems to give them the results they want, but they cannot resist the new products and magical ingredients that hit the market with great fanfare so frequently. When the products do not work, they turn to increasingly invasive treatments, now available at medi-spas and strip malls in your neighborhood.

My approach is different. I teach patients how to achieve profound, long-lasting changes to their skin without having to spend thousands of dollars on the latest products, laser treatments, and peels. I always recommend that my patients give the Lancer Method a try before opting for anything invasive. For many of my patients, my at-home skin care program proves to be intervention enough. They see rapid results and save time, money, and discomfort. I am talking about bringing the science of skin care and anti-aging technology home. The full-body program you will find in *Younger* is state-of-the-art dermatology, and you are in charge. My groundbreaking approach to treating the skin has produced such good results that many patients have delayed or skipped invasive treatments they had been considering.

Of course, your skin reflects your physical and emotional health. If you want to look younger, you have to combat the effects of time by living an anti-aging lifestyle. And in this book I will outline the best lifestyle choices you can make in order to get the best results. After all, making the right choices in all aspects of your life, including diet, exercise, and stress management, is essential if you want to restore the youthful glow to your skin.

Think of this book as an extended visit to my office. You will become an associate patient. I want to show you how to be comfortable in your own skin. I want you to smile at your reflection in the mirror. When you look good, you feel good. And when you feel good, you look even better. My breakthrough anti-aging method will transform you.

Harold Lancer, MD

FELLOW, AMERICAN ACADEMY OF DERMATOLOGY
BEVERLY HILLS, CALIFORNIA

Introduction

The Best Anti-Aging Technique: Harnessing the Skin's Natural Healing Power

Looking your best is serious business. More than thirty years ago, I embarked on a lifelong professional quest to find new ways to repair complexion imperfections. A traumatic and painful event that happened in my childhood lies at the root of my obsession with skin. When I was seven years old, I accidentally fell into a tub of near-boiling water. My brother and I were bundled up, playing catch in the unheated basement of our old farmhouse. My father had just finished bleeding our ancient steam furnace and had left the tub of steaming water to cool. Running backward to catch a ball my brother had thrown, I stumbled and fell into the vat. By the time I was pulled from the searing water, 10 percent of my body had been severely burned. Fortunately, the snowsuit I was wearing saved me from more extensive injuries.

My mother, who emigrated from Austria with the rest of my family after World War II, used Old World remedies to treat the burns. She slathered my raw skin with a poultice made from Crisco, egg yolks, baking soda, and water. She wrapped me in strips of sheets she had torn. I was a mummy.

My rural hometown did not have a burn unit. In fact, we did not even have a hospital nearby. We could not have afforded to go to one anyway. There were no

dermatologists in our Connecticut farm town, just kindly Dr. Jones, a family prac-
titioner and a dead ringer for Christopher Plummer, actor extraordinaire. After
my initial visit, I revisited Dr. Jones's office every day. He cleaned my wounds,
applying Vaseline with a tongue depressor to help them heal, greasing my way
to recovery.

Watching Dr. Jones change the dressing each day, I was impressed by how
meticulous his attention to detail was during the healing process. Weeks went
by as I watched him work with next to nothing. Gradually, my wounds healed.
Except for a small scar on one of my hips, you would never know I had been so
badly burned.

I would never wish a traumatic burn on anyone, let alone a child, but in my
case the unfortunate incident had a life-changing outcome. My very early experience with burns steered me toward my life's work in dermatology. I had always
loved watching my mother in the kitchen as she mixed ingredients when she
baked or cooked. After my dressings were removed, I began to mix potions in
old glass Alka-Seltzer bottles to use as body lotions. I would experiment with my
"products" on my sister's skin in exchange for doing her chores.

Ever since those days in Dr. Jones's office, I have been fascinated by skin—how
it heals, how it ages, how it differs among people, and how skin care has evolved.
Watching my own skin recover from injury helped me develop an incredible sense
of what makes skin beautiful, and inspired me to specialize in repair and healing.
Even with true dermatological disease and cancer, a visibly pleasing cosmetic
end result is of key importance to me. With this intention, one of my specialties
became scar-free skin cancer removal.

I had learned from my own experience that skin has the remarkable capacity
to mend itself. Skin regenerates quickly and efficiently when you are young. As
you age, beginning at about twenty, the repair process slows down, allowing lines,
wrinkles, dullness, and dryness to develop. Harnessing and using that healing
power was clearly the key to restoring the skin's vibrant glow and youthful tone. I
set out to find ways to take advantage of the skin's own healing energy. Whatever
the problem, the answers reside in the physiology of the skin. My unique three-
step anti-aging method was developed over many years in my clinical practice.
The Lancer Method stimulates the skin's underlying mechanisms to work properly to heal and repair the skin in as little as ten minutes a day.

Younger: The Breakthrough Anti-Aging Method for Radiant Skin is a comprehensive
guide to rejuvenating your skin from head to toe. You will learn to maintain your
youthfulness or to reverse the signs of aging with my simple, effective, at-home

program. I will provide a road map to help you navigate the mixed messages—abundantly available now that everyone and his brother thinks and acts as if they are dermatologists. You will learn to see clearly through the maze of misinformation and confusion. I will recommend products that really work. The products can be bought anywhere and on any budget. You may not be aware of the fact that many of the products you own are likely not helping your skin at all. Rather than resorting to invasive procedures to look younger, my program is based on finding the right products and using them in a way that restores your skin. Through years of clinical practice and research, I have discovered that many of the products on the market are not effective in bringing skin back to life. Millions of dollars are wasted on skin care products that do not deliver on the promises made. If you follow my plan, you will get the same transformative results that have brought so many patients to my door.

Part 1 describes the Lancer Method and how it makes skin act younger. We will take a hard look at our culture's youth-obsessed concept of beauty. We have developed unrealistic expectations that drive us to lose our judgment in the search for quick fixes. My program and my practice are rooted in my belief in restoration instead of alteration as the most effective way to have beautiful skin. The Lancer Method taps into the skin's natural healing power. The program's three-step protocol—polish, cleanse, and nourish—is specially designed to maintain your youthful glow or reverse the signs of aging quickly and easily. The Lancer Method is accessible to everyone regardless of budget. I have made three-tiered product recommendations, listing the most effective luxury, moderate, and affordable products and the active ingredients to look for when you are buying skin care products for the program. From your face, neck, and décolletage to your dry, deflated hands, feet, elbows, and knees, the Lancer Method will have you glowing from head to toe. Cellulite, discoloration, scarring, skin tags, thinning hair, brittle nails, and other barnacles of aging will all be addressed—and repaired in no time!

Part 2 begins with "Looking at Your Family Tree," which focuses on the Lancer Ethnicity Scale, a treatment protocol I developed in 1998 that is still in use today. Through clinical research and observation, I discovered that the race, nationality, and global geographic origin of a patient's ancestry are good predictors of the way skin responds to treatments. Failing to consider a patient's heritage can undermine the success of a treatment and may lead to unwanted complications. You will learn how to calculate where you are on the scale and how risky procedures are for your skin tone. We will take the basic Lancer Method a step further for those of you interested in intensive anti-aging skin care. No one likes to look in the mirror and see wrinkles, drooping, bags under the eyes, a sagging jawline, a crepey neck, thin skin, vertical lines above the upper lip, marionette lines at the corners of the mouth, worry lines on the forehead and between the eyes, crow's-feet, aging spots, and broken blood vessels. You will discover what happens to aging skin and how to restore your skin's elasticity and dewy quality. Aging skin requires more nourishment, and my enhanced regimen provides that. This can rejuvenate your complexion and reverse many of the signs of aging. With this supercharged anti-aging regimen, you will see signs of rejuvenation very quickly.

I will also explain how to fine-tune the Lancer Anti-Aging Method for special needs. The number of people affected by acne, rosacea, and sensitive skin is astronomical. They are so involved in dealing with their skin problems that they do not even think about taking action against aging. Since these conditions are so prevalent, I have included in the book an anti-aging program tailored for each of these skin disorders.

Part 3, "The Lancer Anti-Aging Lifestyle," provides pertinent advice on making the right lifestyle choices that support beautiful skin and overall health. Your skin reflects your inner state. Your health, excesses, and emotions are visible in your complexion. Within seconds of meeting a new patient, I can tell whether he or she has been leading a life of excess or is in poor health, often even before the patient is aware that something is wrong. If you are under stress, depressed, not sleeping or eating well, and generally not taking care of yourself, it will show. Bad habits and unhealthy living will add years to your face and the skin on the rest of your body.

Even if you diligently care for your skin, you are going to have trouble achieving results if you do not find a way to lower the stress in your life or to cope with it better. Stress takes a toll on every part of your body. Your skin is no exception. Stress can impair the skin's barrier function, making it easier for irritants to get in and moisture to exit. I will offer suggestions for improving your coping skills and getting more rest and relaxation. Good sleep, after all, is of vital importance to your health and well-being.

I will also talk about how your diet affects your skin. From eliminating processed foods to controlling inflammation, this chapter covers the best way to eat to promote overall health and to give your skin the nourishment it needs to replenish. You may be surprised to hear about some of the "healthy" foods that may be affecting your skin and causing you to look older than you are! My goal in this section is to give you the information you need to improve your digestion, reduce inflammation, and create a balance in your body that will shine through to your skin, taking years off your complexion.

Exercise is essential if you want to be radiant. Physical intimacy is part of the mix. Exercise brings a healthy flush to the skin that indicates an increase in blood circulation. The blood is carrying oxygen and nutrients to the skin, which improves your complexion well beyond those few post-exercise moments. You might be happy to hear that I advocate a measured approach to physical activity. Working out too hard actually can be damaging to your skin. Strenuous exercise promotes inflammation and triggers a cascade of hormones in the same way stress does, prematurely aging the skin. Stretching, yoga, Pilates, and brisk walking, on the other hand, are good for your health and will not damage your skin. I offer an approach to exercise that benefits the body, mind, and skin with some simple workouts designed by my friends to keep you looking and feeling younger.

For those of you who may want to try non-invasive procedures when you feel that you need more than even the best skin care can offer, I cover the latest procedures in the appendixes.

My primary goal in writing this book is to cut through all the hype and confusion surrounding anti-aging procedures and products. When you walk into a cosmetics-oriented office hoping to address a skin problem—anything from wrinkles and lines to sun spots and large pores—you are going to be offered a potpourri of costly invasive or semi-invasive procedures such as injectables, laser resurfacing, and glycolic peels. There are a growing number of options on the menu. I offer every procedure conceivable in my office. They are great for anyone who wants and needs to go the extra mile. But most conditions can be addressed effectively, and I would say more efficiently, with the Lancer Method. Whether you are under twenty-five or somewhat further along in years, this program is not only the first line of defense against aging but also the first line of attack against acne, rosacea, hyperpigmentation, and just about every complexion imperfection. People of all ethnicities and ancestry will respond. Your ongoing commitment to my simple skin care plan will produce great results. Everyone will be asking if you have just returned from vacation or what you have done to look so much younger. Enjoy the attention. You earned it.

YOUNGER

Part One

THE LANCER METHOD

1

The Beauty Trap

We live in a visual age. Everywhere we turn, we are bombarded by provocative images of flawless women and men. Even though it's common knowledge that models all of fourteen years old pose as full-grown women, and that the exquisite pictures in magazines and advertisements have been carefully lit and photo-edited, I continue to see so many people measure themselves against this idealized standard of beauty. Their self-esteem inevitably suffers in a youth-obsessed culture, because they have internalized a standard of beauty that has nothing to do with reality. To make matters worse, cameras are inescapable. Friends and family snap away with their phones and post photos and videos on Facebook and YouTube. The pressure is on. Candid photographs often magnify imperfections, reminding people already critical of themselves that they fall short of their ideal.

Some of the most beautiful people in the world come to my office. I would like to say that they are all confident and secure about their extraordinary looks, but that is far from the truth. Many beauties focus minutely on what is wrong and what needs improvement. The competitive instinct is very intense in all of us, whether or not we are in the public eye. From my patients, I have learned that even people whose faces are admired around the world struggle with the same insecurity and self-criticism as anyone else.

Even Stars Compare

One day, I observed a prominent actress with that Lancer Glow do a barely disguised double take as another longtime patient, a Beverly Hills socialite, came out of a treatment room. The actress was casually dressed and was wearing no makeup at all. She had been texting and happened to look up as the stunning woman walked by. I saw the well-known movie star scrutinize my extravagantly dressed patient from her stilettos to her couture dress to her impressive jewelry. This was how the socialite dressed for everyday life. Though the actress was flawless in her natural beauty, she was in awe. She obviously felt eclipsed by the overall effect of the other woman's appearance, and yet the elegantly dressed woman did not even notice the star's reaction.

The Takeaway: Beauty almost always has a competitive edge, and many people are blind to their own beauty.

If you take good care of yourself mentally and physically, you should be fortunate to live a long, healthy life. As you age, you will want to continue to look as good as you feel. The vast "anti-aging" industry caters to and manages to distort this basic desire. Since the effects of aging are first visible on the skin, dermatology has been elevated to the top of the heap in the war against time. An entire menu of treatments and products exists to minimize the visible signs of aging. This buffet approach to dermatology can provoke impulsive action. Influenced by what their friends have done and the incessant media buzz on the subject, people are driven to buy the latest hyped product and do what they can to look younger. There are plenty of people out there, qualified or not, ready to entice you with unrealistic promises and misleading descriptions of procedures and their aftermath.

The illusion of youth and beauty is sold non-stop everywhere you turn. Exaggerated claims about the latest anti-aging gadget, procedure, serum, and supplement have reshaped consumers' expectations. The media create a fantasy, and consumers respond by demanding faster and faster changes in their appearance. Cosmetics companies, medical spas, surgeons, and procedure-happy "health care providers" and dermatologists have profited by supplying what people have been made to want. There are countless "experts" out there eager to sell you products and procedures that fuel your fantasies.

Medi-Spas: Beware

Do yourself a favor and stay away from medi-spas, as they are called in the trade. Though there might be a medical doctor on staff, a dermatologist or other physician may not be on the premises or even have much to say about the treatment chosen for you. At medi-spas, a medical assistant or a nurse, rather than a board-certified doctor, often makes recommendations for treatments. If you are concerned enough about your face to consider costly and sometimes risky procedures, why would you allow a nurse or aesthetician to determine what is best for you? A medical spa may appear to be less expensive than seeing a board-certified dermatologist, but some bargains will end up costing you more in the long run if you take into account disappointing outcomes as well as the expense of correcting mistakes. It is cost-effective to have a dermatologist, acting as the captain of your anti-aging ship, lead you in reaching a proper plan for reversing the aging process.

QUICK FIXES, MAGIC BULLETS, AND HOPE IN A JAR

People often come to see me in search of a quick fix or reversal. They suffer life-style abuse to their skin or give it minimal care until they have an aha moment, and a light goes on in their heads. The realization that they have neglected to do anything to make themselves look and feel better makes them vulnerable to the anti-aging selling machine. An increasing number of people get hooked on invasive procedures and surgery at a young age. I have met women who had their first face-lift in their thirties. They believe that regular touch-ups will make them ageless. Some have a vision of how they want to look and will make radical changes to their faces and bodies in an attempt to reach an imagined ideal. I have witnessed the cosmetic surgery junkie mentality, and it is disturbing. After the first three procedures, people hooked on surgery lose their compass—and their ability to perceive how they look. They are no longer capable of making a rational judgment. Instead, they keep striving for an elusive vision of perfection.

There is so much noise out there about treatments, products, and procedures, it is hard for most people to cut through the confusion. Many people respond to the hype by buying into the promises and trying whatever they can. Ever hopeful, they go from product to product, treatment to treatment, looking for visible results. Even if they are lucky enough to see improvement, it is usually short-lived.

Some are scared off and decide against any intervention at all, while others are talked into procedures that do not deliver what they expect—or worse, cause problems. I believe in a more measured, realistic approach to skin and beauty. I want you to step back from all the hype and avoid unnecessary procedures. I want you to be in charge of refreshing your skin and making it healthier.

Many patients come to me voicing concern over their age and what it means to be "old." If you are in good shape and look radiant, who cares about how old you are? Age is only a number and a mind-set. True beauty is being the best you can be in all aspects of your life. My goal is to help people recognize and enhance their natural beauty with a little help from many avenues and approaches. To do that, it is important to be realistic about the way you want to look, and patient when achieving the results.

So much energy goes into creating the illusion of beauty. Women come to the office for facials and procedures wearing theatrical-grade makeup, which, of course, we have to remove to examine their skin. Cosmetics are used as camouflage. Rather than correcting problems like uneven pigmentation, big pores, or rosacea, the impulse is to cover up imperfections rather than deal with them. "I couldn't be seen without makeup!" and "I never go out without my face on" are common refrains these days. One of my patients comes for her appointments with a professional makeup artist, who waits in the reception area to reapply her "face" after her treatments. It puzzles me that she spends time and money on her skin, which she never shows to the world in its natural state. My hope is that by following my at-home regimen, your skin will look so good that you will only need to wear minimal makeup, or even none at all.

Whenever I walk into a treatment room to consult with patients, I hand them a mirror and have them point with a Q-tip to what is bothering them. I ask them, "What can I do for you?" I can rarely predict what the response will be. Often the patient's assessment is different from what strikes me at first glance. One person might be bothered by a small blemish on the left side of his outer eye and ignore the skin cancer on the tip of his nose. Another might have excessively pumped-up lips but be worried about a small discoloration under her chin. Insecurity makes people overanalytical about their looks. They become preoccupied with real or imagined defects and obsessive about cosmetic concerns.

Your own self-image is the key to beauty. If you are confident, full of life, and passionate, you will be irresistible; you are more than what you see in the mirror. If you are self-conscious, insecure, and trying too hard, you will telegraph your poor self-image to everyone in countless unspoken ways. If you feel good about yourself, people will respond positively to you. Self-acceptance and confidence are the foundation of beauty—and sex appeal.

Both the subliminal and the obvious messages of the beauty trap are designed to make you dissatisfied with your looks—and to make you go to great lengths and expense to change them. That being said, there is nothing wrong with wanting to improve your appearance. I have spent my life helping men and women to do just that. It is all a matter of degree and expectations. We do get older, after all; everything in nature ages. Though now we can slow down the process and diminish many of the visible signs of aging, many people go too far. Frozen features, duck-bill lips, and skin that is stretched too thin and too tight are alarming, artificial, and draw attention to their attempts to be someone they are not.

I believe in what I call a revolutionary evolution in our thinking about beauty. I have found that rehabilitation works better than surgery and other aggressive treatments to restore the skin's youthful appearance. Though it is simple, my approach is a breakthrough in skin care for the restoration of a healthy, more youthful appearance. You can rejuvenate your skin with the program in this book. You will begin with my breakthrough three-step regimen and combine it with lifestyle changes that prevent further damage and provide an environment in which natural restoration can occur. You will be amazed by the results. You can choose to age gracefully. As people abandon extreme treatments and surgeries to change their looks, our idea of beauty will evolve to be more natural and age-appropriate without sacrificing the vibrancy and appeal of youth.

SIX DIMENSIONS

To be outstanding at my work, I have to think in six dimensions. All people have the obvious three dimensions of length, width, and depth. Time, the fourth, is the overall winning dimension. Time inevitably changes everything. You can try to postpone, delay, or cancel, but time's passing is a reality of life. The fifth dimension is perception: understanding what patients see when they look at their reflections in the mirror, how they perceive themselves. The sixth dimension is the future, and what I can do now that will serve a patient later.

Putting this in more concrete terms, when I consult with a patient, I assess the physical condition of his or her skin and whether it shows signs of aging or disease in three dimensions. Then I have to project into time, imagining what that face will look like ten years from now. All of my patients think in the fifth dimension. They come to see me because they perceive problems. They identify the "flaws" they want me to correct. Their perception of how they look is so often different from what I see. Some discover the slightest sign of aging on close examination and are desperate to stop the process. They either dread or cannot conceive of how they will look as they age. They want to make time disappear. I try to make

Three Women

In a single day, I saw three new female patients at various stages in life. Their stories represent a range of skin care mistakes.

One executive in her late fifties had been a stunning beauty in her heyday but started with radical procedures early on. She did not want her seductive looks to change. As time went by and the procedures piled up, she lost her perception of how she really looked. She had huge, puffy lips, and her entire face and neck were bloated and swollen. The scar tissue from her various surgeries and treatments blocked the lymphatic drainage in her face. Nothing can be done to reverse this condition. A beautiful woman had become the victim of her own fantasy of beauty. I do not know what she sees when she looks in the mirror, but she seems unaware of what she has done to herself. She continues to tweak this and that to prop up her damaged skin. I am now thinking of procedures to help her.

The second woman is a great beauty, very much in the public eye. She is in her late thirties, and her glamorous face is everywhere. Her story is a case of cosmetic illusion. She is unaware of what is happening under all her daily makeup, which leaves her skin dehydrated and uneven. Relying on beauty professionals to apply her makeup, she does not have a true sense of the condition of her skin.

She has no interest in taking the time now to care for her skin. She will not sit still for the least invasive of treatments and is impatient about following a daily regimen. If she continues with this attitude, she is going to see her skin change in ways she cannot ignore. In ten years, she will have to take drastic measures to restore her skin's quality. If she started with a balanced skin care program now, she could save herself future grief and keep her skin looking young for many more years. Everyone in my office will work with me to convince her that this is the right time to do something to save her lovely face.

The last woman, an actress at the height of her beauty at thirty, is perplexed. She came to see me to get ready for a big red-carpet event and did not know what she should be doing to take care of her skin or where to start. I was able to explain the importance of home care to her and the science behind the Lancer Method. Not only will she see an immediate improvement in her skin, but her home care routine will keep her skin looking young and fresh.

The Takeaway: Surgery and invasive procedures can make you lose touch with how you really look. Take steps early to care for your skin at home before you need to take more drastic measures.

my patients realistic about the passage of time. We all get older. The goal is to do the job well.

I am a minimalist when it comes to creating a treatment plan. Rather than jumping right in with an invasive approach, I begin with skin care and then determine the least invasive route to take that will satisfy a particular patient's need. I avoid the quick-fix approach, and make sure I have a full understanding of where my patient lies on the Lancer Ethnicity Scale, a classification system I developed that gauges how a patient's skin will react to various treatments based on ancestry. I then devise the best course of action possible. My patients become active participants in a plan to look and feel their best. I am writing this book so that you will have the tools and the knowledge to do the same. There have been so many advances in procedures to make your complexion look younger. The trick is to find the right path. Rather than offering you a recipe or a menu for making extreme changes to your appearance, I want you to learn how to evaluate your looks realistically. You will have the savvy to reject the promises of the deceptive beauty trap, adjust your expectations, and remain radiantly beautiful and appealing for the rest of your life.

AGING IS FIRST VISIBLE ON YOUR SKIN

Exposed to the world, your skin shows the first signs of aging. You react to what you see in the mirror, but you probably do not realize that the aging of your skin directly reflects what is happening to your physical brain and the way it functions. Skin and brain cells develop from the same tissue, called the ectoderm, which is the outermost layer of an embryo. The nervous system, epidermis, nails, hair, and glands of the skin are all formed from the ectoderm as the embryo develops. If your skin is aging prematurely, your brain is undergoing parallel changes. When you are diligent about improving your skin—and a big part of that is lifestyle—the benefits will reach far beyond your appearance. The lifestyle changes you make will keep your brain functioning at optimal levels, boost your energy, and lift your spirits.

You are undoubtedly all too familiar with the visible signs of aging—thinning, sagging, fragile, dull, wrinkled skin with dark spots in sun-exposed areas. Though these signs may occur at different rates in different patients, they are unavoidable if you do nothing to prevent them. Genetics, environmental factors, nutrition, stress, and sun exposure all contribute to the aging of your skin.

Visible Aging by Decade

If left unchecked, skin undergoes a predictable series of changes with age. With proper attention, you can slow the process down, erase some damage, and start over with a much-improved overall complexion from head to toe. Here is what to expect decade by decade.

Twenties: Biological shifts begin but usually do not show yet. For example, hormone levels begin to decline from their peaks in adolescence. The twenties are the age of prevention. During this decade, most skin problems are the result of a lack of skin care and a party lifestyle, including smoking, excessive alcohol consumption, poor diet, not enough sleep, and stress.

Thirties: The skin begins to show signs of aging. Laugh lines, crow's-feet, skin laxity, and uneven color can start to appear. The complexion becomes drier, duller, and lacks luster.

Forties: This is the decade when skin quality can change significantly. The production line of repair is faulty. The buildup of old skin cells blocks natural radiance. The loss of collagen and elastin can be seen in drooping eyelids, a softening jawline, and a crepey neck. Age spots appear on the back of the hands and face. Hair starts to turn gray.

Fifties: Since the padding of fat beneath the skin has diminished, the face has more angles and hollows. The reduction of underlying fat leads to loss of firmness in the hands and neck. The fat that remains can form distortion under the eyes. Bone loss affects the facial bones, which shrink from the skin, resulting in sagging muscle mass and loose skin. The upper lip thins, and the lower lip becomes more pronounced. Hormonal changes take root in both genders. Cumulative environmental exposure contributes to wrinkling, drooping, and unevenness in skin tone. Hair can appear where you do not want it and thin where you do.

Sixties: Poor circulation can rob the skin of vitality. Since the skin is increasingly thin and dry, it becomes more sensitive and prone to irritation. Wrinkles deepen and gravity does its work. Ears elongate and jowls form. Wounds take much longer to heal, because skin repairs itself more slowly.

How much you decide to intervene with this process is up to you. The course of action will depend on when you begin and what you want to achieve. *Younger* will give you the tools to improve your skin and provides you with the background you need to weed out the truth from the hype. The first step, no matter what your age, is to establish a home-based program and stick with it. As you will learn, the Lancer Method is unique, and with it you can see results in just days. The improvements will surprise you, I promise.

WHAT CAUSES SKIN TO AGE

The changes in your skin are a consequence of genetically programmed internal aging, which occurs with time; extrinsic aging, caused by environmental factors such as sun exposure, which causes photo-aging; and lifestyle. Intrinsic, biological aging involves internal changes at the cellular level. In the most general sense, the reproduction of skin cells slows down as you age. As you get older, your body produces more enzymes that break down collagen and elastic tissue, the bundles of protein that give skin its plumpness and bounce. Finally, the material that fills the spaces surrounding cells, called the extracellular matrix, diminishes, because the rate at which it is formed slows down. The matrix provides structural support for the cells, and when the volume of the extracellular matrix decreases, the cells collapse on one another, causing the skin to lose tone. Falling levels of hormones, especially estrogen and testosterone, play a part in the aging process as well. Exposure to environmental factors—like sun, cold, pollutants, toxins—ages your skin from the outside. The older you are, the longer you have been exposed to harmful influences. Diet, exercise, sleep habits, stress levels, and illness affect the internal processes that age you. All this shows up on your face. You are your skin.

The patients I have seen who have not been blessed with good health, whose medical histories include serious physical ailments, almost always show signs of premature aging. Their skin can look pasty, pale, and dull. I work with multiple medical specialists to cooperate on the process of internal and external repair for medically challenged patients. My at-home skin routine has restored the health and vitality of their skin by improving the cycle of cell renewal and self-repair.

10 WAYS TO AGE YOUR SKIN PREMATURELY

A number of things you do or fail to do are known skin agers. The following list contains the biggest offenses. You stand a good chance of looking older and damaging your skin if you:

1. **Do not have a good daily skin care regimen.**

   Taking care of your skin should be as routine as brushing your teeth. You go to the dentist regularly for exams and cleanings. Your skin deserves at least as much attention as your teeth. You need to polish, clean, and nourish your skin each day with products that will keep it healthy and clear. My program will show you how. Make a point of seeing a dermatologist to discuss good overall maintenance and to plan a treatment program, starting with non-invasive procedures to keep your skin looking young.

2. **Fail to use sunscreen every day.**

Sun exposure without protection is the most damaging thing you can do to your skin. Use a sunscreen of at least 30 SPF on your skin every day. My protocol for when and how often to apply appears below. Remember to wear sunglasses when you are outdoors. Squinting can cause crow's-feet and frown lines, not to mention damage to your vision. Here are some additional tips to remember:

- Limit your time outdoors when the sun is at its peak between 10:00 a.m. and 3:00 p.m.
- Give your skin time to absorb sunscreen before sun exposure. Apply sunscreen liberally, fifteen minutes to half an hour before going outdoors.
- Use enough sunscreen to coat all skin that will not be covered by clothing. Most people apply only 25 to 50 percent of the recommended amount. Follow the guideline of "one ounce, enough to fill a shot glass" to cover the exposed areas of your body.
- Do not forget your lips. Use a product that has been specially formulated for your lips with an SPF of 20 or more.
- Wear long pants, a shirt with long sleeves, and a hat with a wide brim if you are planning to be out during peak hours. The lighter the color and more tightly woven your clothes, the more protection from the sun they will afford. A white T-shirt has an SPF of only 5. You can buy clothing with built-in SPF or wash the clothing you wear outdoors with a laundry aid like SunGuard, which gives clothes a higher SPF.
- Reapply sunscreen frequently, every two or three hours, depending on the time of day and what you are doing. Be sure to use a generous amount each time. A thin coat of protection can reduce the effectiveness by as much as 50 percent. Remember to protect your ears and hairline.
- Be careful about reflected light. A beach umbrella or shade trees give you only moderate protection. UV rays reflect from sand, snow, and concrete. They even penetrate water. The underpart of your chin is particularly vulnerable to reflected light. You do not want to contribute to signs of aging on your neck if you can prevent it.

- There is no such thing as a healthy tan. If a burnished look appeals to you anyway, take it slowly and let the skin build up melanin gradually. Do not use tanning beds. Tanning beds and sunlamps generally emit 93 to 99 percent UVA radiation. This is three times the UVA radiation given off by the sun.
- Be aware that some medications increase the risk of UV ray damage. Check with your doctor about the medications you are taking and any new ones that might be prescribed.
- Know that some skin types are at a greater risk of UV damage.

3. **Smoke or are exposed to secondhand smoke for long periods of time.**

Cigarette smoke—even secondhand—triggers biochemical changes that accelerate aging. The damage can be seen under a microscope for smokers as young as twenty. People who smoke are more likely to develop deeply wrinkled, leathery skin with a yellow tinge. Smoking depletes the body of vitamin C, a key anti-oxidant that helps to keep your skin plump and moist. Some believe that smoking is as damaging to skin as UVA rays. The good news is that you can improve your skin tone if you stop.

4. **Drink too much alcohol.**

Drinking liquor affects your circulation. Small blood vessels dilate and blood flows near the surface, creating a flushed appearance. Alcohol is a diuretic that dehydrates the entire body, as is evidenced by the intense thirst of a hangover. When your skin is dehydrated, it becomes scaly and taut with superficial lines and premature aging. Dehydration becomes more prevalent with age. Drinking will only intensify the problem. A glass or two of red wine with dinner now and then is not a problem. Regular, habitual, excessive drinking is. Make sure to drink plenty of water whenever you drink alcoholic beverages.

5. **Are a couch potato.**

Moderate exercise is an important part of anti-aging skin care. Exercise increases circulation and blood flow to the skin, stimulates neurons, and produces sweat that cleans the body from the inside. Increased circulation carries more oxygen and nutrients to the skin. More natural oils are produced that keep your skin looking healthy. Exercise keeps your muscles strong and firm, and muscles support your skin, giving it a smooth appearance. Most important, exercise is a stress buster that helps you to relax. Warning: Working out too intensely can be harmful. Not only does an extreme workout produce stress hormones, but it will create free radicals as well.

6. **Eat processed, junk, and fried foods, along with too many simple carbs.**

   Processed food is dead food: It has lost most of its important nutrients in processing. The natural nutrients that are lost are often replaced by synthetic additives—and then there are the toxic preservatives, food colors, and other chemicals. Processed food is loaded with sugar and salt, both of which are bad for your skin. To look younger, you need to eat more whole and raw foods. Fatty, greasy, and oily foods made with saturated fats, trans fats, and hydrogenated oil become toxic when heated and create free radicals. Simple carbohydrates—all the white foods, including bread, rice, pasta, sweets, and most desserts—are digested quickly and turned into sugar. All that sugar sets off glycation, which accelerates the aging process. When sugar comes in contact with collagen, an immediate chemical reaction occurs. Free radicals and advanced glycation end products, appropriately called AGEs, are formed. AGEs damage the protein fibers of collagen and elastin and signal inflammatory processes in the cells. If you can reduce glycation through a clean, plant-based diet, you can slow the aging process.

7. **Engage in yo-yo dieting or weight cycling.**

   The starve-and-binge cycle, known as weight cycling, is very damaging to your skin, especially if a lot of weight is involved. Repeated stretching by gaining weight may damage your skin's elasticity; conversely, losing weight too fast can leave your skin saggy. Yo-yo dieting also throws your hormones out of balance, increasing production of the stress hormone cortisol. Too much cortisol causes inflammation, which ages you.

8. **Fail to get enough quality sleep or experience "sleep interruptus."**

   As you already know, most likely from your own experience, sleep loss can lead to dull skin, dark circles under the eyes, and eventually fine lines. When you do not get enough sleep, your body releases more of the stress hormone cortisol. In addition to causing inflammation, cortisol breaks down collagen. When you have inadequate sleep, your body releases too little human growth hormone, which declines as you age anyway. HGH works during the night to repair tissue, restoring skin cells after the wear and tear of the day. If you are not getting enough sleep, you are preventing the repair process from being effective.

9. **Stress out chronically, with a mind that will not quit.**

Stress causes eczema, hives, rosacea, and psoriasis, and there is a strong connection with acne. Stress disturbs your body's homeostasis and throws your hormones out of whack. Cortisol levels stay elevated, which creates free radicals and impairs the rejuvenation of your skin. Emotional stress retards cell renewal, destroys collagen fibers in the skin, and breaks down elastin. Your skin's barrier protection can weaken when you are under stress, which affects skin hydration and your immune system. More pathogens are able to invade your body through the compromised barrier. This breakdown is part of the reason why you might get sick during times of stress. Unrelenting stress can result in the thinning and dulling of your hair as well.

Oprah asked me to work with twenty women in the last season of her *Oprah Winfrey Show*. Every one of them had significant personal problems and hardship. Several women were in serious financial trouble, many had bad marriages, one was divorced and raising a handicapped child alone, another was dealing with the suicide of a child, a few had children who had overdosed, and several had to care for aged parents. Though they were sophisticated about skin care and aware of what they needed to do to stay healthy, they were overwhelmed by the difficult circumstances in their lives. They were focused on family disruptions and daily struggles, and they no longer bothered to maintain themselves.

Their lives were so stressful that they did not think about what was good for them. They could not take a step back to consider what the unchecked stress was doing to their bodies. They had let themselves go. Skin changes are gradual, and then, there they are. These women did not like the changes they were seeing, but they felt hopeless about addressing them. Oprah brought me in to show them what they could do themselves with little time or expense. They needed a program they could easily incorporate into their lives.

When they began my self-care program, their skin responded within three to five days. They had dramatic results by using my polish-cleanse-nourish method to rejuvenate their skin. We added facials and some non-invasive treatments to show them how far they could go to reverse the signs of aging without extreme measures. The improvements extended beyond their appearance. When their skin brightened up, so did they. They were energized and better able to handle the hardship in their lives. They realized they deserved to give themselves the same care that they did not hesitate to give to others. The changes in how they looked and felt buoyed them up. They understood that taking care of themselves had to be a priority.

10. **Sleep every night with your face on your pillow in the same position.**

If you sleep on your side every night, your cheek, jawline, and neck are pushed against the pillow. Your skin could be folded or creased for several hours a night. Over the years, those folds become etched into your skin to form sleep lines. Sleeping in the fetal position not only affects your face, but could make your décolletage crepey. A facedown position may cause wrinkles in your forehead. Sleeping on your back is the best way to go. There is no pressure on your face, and you breathe more oxygen.

This list is not meant as a reprimand. There are very few people who do not abuse themselves in one way or another. I will use myself as an example. I religiously follow the anti-aging lifestyle that I recommend to my patients. Though I eat well and exercise just about every day, I get up at 4:30 a.m., a learned habit from surgical days. I am at the office five days a week from 7:00 a.m. to 7:00 p.m. and usually show up on Saturday. I turn in early at night. My wife has a hard time getting me to take a vacation. I love what I do but have to acknowledge that working so hard is addictive behavior. With all that I know about the body and aging, I still follow an extremely demanding schedule and do not build in enough downtime to relax. I tell you this to make it clear that no one is perfect. We all neglect ourselves in one way or another. If I have convinced you to try to break your bad habits, take them on one at a time. If you ease into changing your behavior, you will have a better chance at success.

CELL AGING AND YOUR LIFESTYLE CHOICES

The natural degeneration associated with aging occurs in your DNA, which holds the genetic or hereditary material that makes you who you are. A chromosome is a long strand of DNA, consisting of protein and tight coils of DNA. The tips of chromosomes are protected by caps called telomeres, which prevent coils of DNA in our chromosomes from unraveling and fraying. Our cells are constantly dividing, supplying new, healthy cells that function properly to keep our bodies running well. Each time a cell divides, the telomeres get shorter and become less effective at protecting the chromosomes from injury and deterioration. If you think of a telomere as the tip at the end of a shoelace, you will get the idea. A shoelace begins to unravel when the tip wears down. When telomeres become too short, essential parts of the DNA can be damaged. Eventually, the cell is no longer able to divide and replicate, and it dies. In effect, a telomere acts as a timer on the life of a cell.

The aging of your cells does not always match your chronological age. Scientists can use the length of a cell's telomeres to determine its age and how many more times it will replicate. The way you live affects the rate at which your telomeres shorten. Your telomeres can be worn down by an unhealthy lifestyle. Prematurely short telomeres have been linked to obesity, a deficient diet, and a sedentary lifestyle.

DO HORMONES KEEP YOU YOUNG?

The lowering of natural hormone levels over time is another factor in the skin's intrinsic aging process. The hormones most involved with your skin include estrogen, progesterone, testosterone, DHEA, and human growth hormone. When the levels of these hormones fall as you age, particularly with menopause, your skin is significantly affected.

Estrogen

Estrogen allows the skin to remain plump and wrinkle-free. By maintaining the fluid balance, this hormone keeps the skin moist. Although estrogen receptors in skin are located all over the body, they are concentrated in the face. These receptors support collagen production. When estrogen levels go down, so does the number of receptors.

The decrease in estrogen during perimenopause and menopause is a major factor in aging. Estrogen maintains the thickness of the outer layer of skin. When estrogen levels decline, the skin thins. Estrogen loss causes hot flashes, during which the skin becomes flushed and blotchy. Estrogen has anti-inflammatory properties. The inflammation of the skin and in the body increases as production of the hormone slows down and eventually stops. The precipitous drop in estrogen levels during menopause means a reduction in collagen production and breaking down of existing collagen, which leads to a loss of firmness.

Progesterone

Progesterone, another female hormone that decreases with age, reduces inflammation and stimulates collagen production. This hormone regulates sleep and boosts immunity and brain function. When progesterone levels decline during perimenopause, such symptoms as poor sleep, mood swings, and foggy thinking can occur. The sleep disruption many women experience during menopause is tied to falling progesterone levels.

Getting the proper amount of restorative sleep is essential if you want to keep your skin looking young and fresh.

Testosterone

The chief male hormone or androgen is testosterone. Testosterone is involved in the production of sebum, an oily substance secreted by the sebaceous glands in the skin. On the upside, sebum helps reduce wrinkles. Male skin takes longer to wrinkle because of the level of testosterone in men's bodies. On the downside, too much sebum contributes to acne.

Following menopause, the balance between estrogen and androgens is thrown off. This can lead to adult acne in women. In addition, the relative increase in androgens can cause other male characteristics to appear in women, including facial hair and pattern baldness. Testosterone contributes to mood, energy, sex drive, muscle mass, and memory in men and women. As testosterone levels fall, these qualities recede in both sexes. Lower testosterone also affects weight management.

DHEA

DHEA, a precursor hormone to estrogen and androgens, protects against obesity by shifting metabolism from fat storage to energy burning. DHEA supports the dermis and increases the production of collagen. It protects against oxidative stress, which is a very important anti-aging function.

Human Growth Hormone

Human growth hormone (HGH) has become the magic bullet of the moment. Used by weight lifters for some time to build muscles, HGH is being pushed by supplement companies as a miracle anti-aging agent. As the name indicates, HGH enhances tissue growth, increases muscle mass, and strengthens bone density. When HGH declines, your skin loses elasticity and your body loses muscle, which makes for saggy skin.

EVERYTHING RUSTS WITH AGE

Free radicals are a by-product of your metabolism, created when your cells produce energy. Almost all of the oxygen you breathe is used for this purpose. The remaining oxygen molecules lose electrons, and those molecules become free radicals, also known as ROS (reactive oxygen species). These unstable molecules are like vampires that attack normal molecules to steal the electrons that they are missing. Seeking to stabilize themselves, free radicals attack the fatty membrane of a cell or the DNA within the nucleus to appropriate electrons. Once the free radical steals electrons from its victim, the free radical is neutralized, but the victim becomes a new free radical, as if bitten by a vampire. That free radical steals electrons to stabilize itself, and a chain reaction begins. Think of slices of apple left out on a plate. The apple turns brown. This is oxidation made visible. The same process is at work when metal rusts or tarnishes. In nature, everything eventually breaks down, and the human body is no different.

Many environmental factors speed the formation of free radicals, most notably exposure to the sun's damaging ultraviolet rays, a subject of importance I will discuss at length later. Free radicals are produced during the normal metabolism of food. Certain foods have a high potential for setting off a destructive cascade of free radicals. For example, foods that are fried at a high temperature can cause fat molecules to become unstable. Toxic heavy metals like mercury, aluminum, lead, and cadmium create free radicals. Hormones like cortisol that are created when you are stressed also produce a free radical cascade. If free radical production goes out of control, inflammation results.

When it comes to your skin, free radicals are trouble. They attack the fats and proteins in the skin and severely damage skin cells, causing premature aging. The good news is that you can minimize free radical damage with simple lifestyle changes. You can replenish anti-oxidants with topical applications, supplements, and your diet. For instance, vitamins A, C, and E are anti-oxidants that slow the aging process by preventing free radicals from oxidizing other molecules.

Too Much of a Good Time

One of my patients, the daughter of a legendary musician, brought her best friend from England to see me. Her very attractive friend was in her late twenties, but had been living the high life since she was twelve, a glamorous fixture on the party circuit for fifteen or sixteen years. Her jet-set life was taking a toll on her appearance. She had spent too much time sunning on yachts in the South of France, and her skin suffered for it. Late nights filled with tobacco and alcohol consumption were beginning to show. Her pores were enlarged, and her freshness was fading. Her story shows that even the genetically blessed can age prematurely if they neglect themselves. She came to me because she knew she had to clean up her act.

Her lifestyle was quickly catching up with her. She was certain that her looks were slipping away. Younger women were replacing her in the spotlight, and she was convinced that she was about to be discarded from her world. She was wired and anxious, and her emotional state was driving her to greater excesses. Her life was spinning out of control.

Skin care was all that was required to reverse the visible effects of her self-destructive lifestyle, but she clearly needed more than that. If she did not take steps to break bad habits and change her life, she would be in trouble physically and psychologically. I was able to convince her that she needed help with a lot more than her appearance. I referred her to my team of multi-specialty doctors for medical rehabilitation to help her make a clean break with her old lifestyle.

The Takeaway: Adopting a healthier lifestyle is like pressing the rewind button on time.

EXTRINSIC AGING

The condition of your skin stems more directly from how you treat it than from your biological programming. The environment you create in your body can speed up or slow down the intrinsic aging process. What you eat, especially your consumption of alcohol and sugar, how much you sleep, your tobacco use, the level of stress in your life, anxiety, and depression—all play a role in how you age. You have to make healthy choices if you want to delay the aging process. When you learn about the effects that your behavior and habits have on your skin, I hope you will want to change your ways. Understanding how some of your habits put the intrinsic aging processes into overdrive is an important first step. Learning how to stimulate cell renewal with the Lancer Method is another.

You now have an overview of what makes you age, both inside and out. You know the habits that will push you toward premature aging and accelerate the visible signs of skin aging. The next chapter probes more deeply into how the skin restores itself. Manipulating this mechanism is at the core of the Lancer Method.

2

The Skin's Natural Process of Renewal

Your skin is constantly refreshing itself by producing new cells and sloughing off dead ones. The cycle takes twenty-eight days when you are young. As you age, cell renewal gradually slows down. By the time you are fifty, the process takes twice as long as it did when you were in your twenties. Old cells are more vulnerable to the internal processes of aging. The Lancer Method is based on the principle that if you stimulate the skin's built-in repair system, you can reverse some of the visible signs of aging and slow down the rate of future damage. If you back up your skin care program with an anti-aging lifestyle, you will weaken the forces that drive biological aging while you harness your skin's own healing power.

As you will see, the skin is made up of three layers: epidermis, dermis, and subcutaneous tissue. Most anti-aging regimens and products focus solely on the dermis, and that is why they do not give you the results you are hoping for. My thirty years of clinical experience have shown that you must treat the epidermis to rejuvenate and repair the skin, specifically the stratum corneum. Without this crucial step, no regimen or product will work. Now, before we explore exactly how to treat the skin, it is important for you to understand the skin's structure and how it renews itself.

Looks Like a Teenager

I have a patient whose age is impossible to guess. Though she is in her late forties, you would think she was in her teens if she wore her hair in pigtails. A green-eyed blonde of mixed Northern European heritage, she has transcended expectations for her fair skin type. Her fair skin should show age early and easily, yet it has remained tight and fresh.

She is a former ballerina, so there may have been some nutritional deficiencies early on in her life. A dancer's need to be pencil-thin typically leads to abuse of her body with starvation diets and cigarettes. I do not know how this woman behaved as a dancer, but I do know how well she takes care of herself now.

This patient has been a devotee of the Lancer Method for sixteen years and has shown extraordinary discipline in taking good care of herself with skin hygiene and an anti-aging lifestyle. She has been using the Lancer Method since I initially developed it and does not skip a day of her skin care routine. Genetics are only partially responsible for her youthful appearance. She has avoided the visible signs of aging by consistently stimulating her skin to be radiant with her at-home regime.

The Takeaway: Skin care and healthy living can trump genetics.

SKIN REFRESHER COURSE

Most people think of their skin as a simple outer covering rather than the complex, vital organ that it is. It's easy to take skin for granted, focusing on how it looks and being unaware of all that it does. Your skin is the largest organ of your body, makes up 15 percent of your body weight, and covers a total area of about twenty square feet. It offers the first line of defense against the external environment, acting as a protective shield from light, heat, injury, and infection. Skin operates as a two-way protective barrier that prevents microbes and harmful environmental elements from entering your body, and prevents water from exiting. Among its many other functions, the skin regulates body temperature, stores water and fat, and operates as a sensory organ that permits the sensations of touch and heat. Skin gathers and communicates sensory information that stimulates an immune response to protect you from disease. Skin plays a major role in your overall health.

Your skin is an entire community with a variety of different cells, blood vessels, nerves, muscles that make hair stand up, and an intricate communication system. If you want to look younger, you have to understand the anatomy of the skin.

The skin consists of three layers. The epidermis, the outer layer, plays a big role in the Lancer Method. Below the epidermis is the middle layer of skin, called the dermis; the layer beneath that is called subcutaneous tissue or the hypodermis. Let's examine how these layers interact.

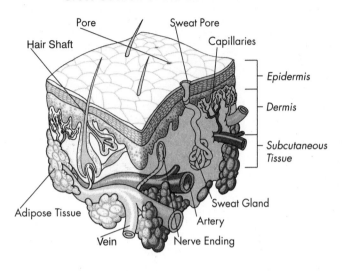

Cross Section of the Skin

The Hypodermis or Subcutaneous Layer

Starting from the deepest layer and moving up to the surface, we will first examine the hypodermis. This level is a network of collagen, connective tissue, and fat cells. The subcutaneous layer houses larger blood vessels and nerves that bring nourishment and sensation to the skin. Containing about 50 percent of the body's fat, this layer varies in thickness from person to person. The subcutaneous tissue conserves body heat and acts as a shock absorber to protect your organs from injury. The hypodermis attaches the skin to the underlying bones and muscles.

Aging Changes in the Hypodermis

- As you age, this layer of subcutaneous fat thins.
- Consequently, you have less natural insulation, which reduces your body's ability to maintain body temperature and increases your risk of injury.
- The fat layer absorbs some medications, including some anti-anxiety drugs. A reduction of this layer can change how the medications work.
- Thinning of the layer of subcutaneous fat can make the face gaunt or skeletal.

The Dermis

There are many special cells and structures located in the middle layer, the dermis, which contains blood vessels, lymph vessels, hair follicles, sweat glands, sebaceous oil glands, scent glands, and the nerves responsible for the sensations of pain, itchiness, and temperature. Collagen, composed of bundles of protein, is the main component of the dermis and the most abundant protein in the body. The dermis is held together by collagen and elastin, another protein. These proteins keep your skin supple and resilient. Collagen fibers give support to the skin, and elastin provides flexibility and strength. Elastin gives your skin the bounce to return to its original position when pinched or poked. Collagen and elastin break down with age. When this happens, your skin loses volume and begins to sag and wrinkle.

The top level of the dermis is called the papillary region. The finger-like projections from this region extend to the epidermis and strengthen the connection between the two layers of skin. In the papillary region collagen is perpendicular to the skin's surface and elastin is horizontal, forming a latticework. The reticular region below is thicker and dense with collagen and elastin. Both types of fibers are arranged parallel to the surface of the skin in this layer.

Aging Changes in the Dermis

- The reduction of collagen and elastin caused by aging affects the strength and elasticity of skin. This is especially visible in areas exposed to the sun. Leathery, weatherworn skin is the result.
- The number of blood vessels is reduced, and those that remain become more fragile, resulting in bruising and bleeding under the skin.
- Capillaries collapse, creating red spider veins on the hands and face.
- The sebaceous glands produce less sebum, resulting in dryness and itchiness. This effect tends to begin for women after menopause and not until eighty for men.
- Hair thins, because the number of hair follicles diminishes.
- The sweat glands are not as productive, which makes it more difficult for your body to keep cool.
- Free radicals can damage fats and proteins in dermal cells, which leads to premature aging.

Most anti-aging and skin care programs try to fight aging by targeting the dermis, the location of collagen and elastin production. My skin care program instead focuses on the epidermis, particularly its outermost layer, and the stratum corneum. I have discovered that if you want to effect significant change, the dermis is not where the action is.

The dermis interacts with the epidermis via a signaling system that not only stimulates the immune system but also promotes the repair and remodeling of skin when injured. The Lancer Method uses this signaling system to restore your skin.

The Basement Membrane or the Dermal/Epidermal Junction

This porous membrane allows and controls the exchange of cells and fluid between the dermis and the epidermis. Holding the two layers together, the membrane is a highly irregular connection that undulates, increasing the surface area over which nutrients, oxygen, and waste products can be exchanged. The basement membrane has an important function in skin rejuvenation, because it regulates cell migration, an important process of regeneration that occurs in the epidermis.

Aging Changes in the Basement Membrane

- The boundary between the epidermis and the dermis flattens out with age, which slows down the exchange between the two levels.

- Photo-aging accelerates this flattening, resulting in decreased transfer of nutrients between layers.

The Epidermis

We will examine the epidermis closely, because its actions are highly important to the Lancer Method. As you can see in the illustration on page 28, the outer layer of skin is composed of either four or five layers, depending on the location of the skin. From the bottom up, they are: the basal or germinal layer (stratum basale); the spinous layer (stratum spinosum); the granular layer (stratum granulosum); the clear layer (stratum lucidum), a translucent layer found only on the lips, palms, and soles of the feet; and the cornified or horny layer (stratum corneum). We are most concerned with the top layer, the cornified layer, for reasons I will explain.

Layers of the Epidermis

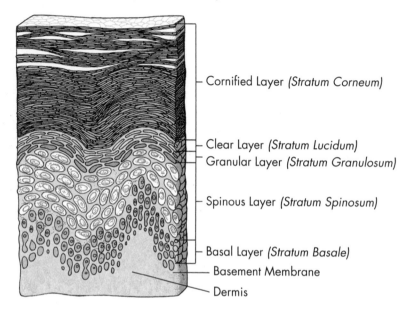

Cornified Layer *(Stratum Corneum)*

Clear Layer *(Stratum Lucidum)*
Granular Layer *(Stratum Granulosum)*

Spinous Layer *(Stratum Spinosum)*

Basal Layer *(Stratum Basale)*
Basement Membrane
Dermis

Basal Layer

The basal layer contains Merkel cells, which are believed to be involved in the sensations we feel through our skin. Melanocytes are also found in the bottom layer of the epidermis. Those cells produce melanin, a brown pigment that gives skin its color and protects against ultraviolet rays.

The basal cells continually divide to form new keratinocytes that replace old cells, which are shed from the skin's surface. Keratinocytes produce keratin, a long thread-like protein that makes the skin strong and has a protective role. Keratinocytes, which are shaped like columns, attach to the basement membrane zone. These cells divide and make the cells that move up to the outer layers of the epidermis.

Spinous Layer

The spinous layer is responsible for vitamin D synthesis. Langerhans cells found in this layer are the immune system's front line of defense. As the new cells move through this layer, they become flatter.

Granular Layer

As they move through the spinous and granular layers, keratinocytes become increasingly flatter and their nuclei begin to degenerate. In this layer, they become cells composed of granules that are filled with proteins that promote hydration to keep the skin moist. The cells secrete a "cement" made of fats, fatty acids, and cholesterol, which fills the spaces between the cells and increases cohesion, making the epidermis an effective waterproof barrier.

Cornified Layer

By the time the granular cells reach the cornified layer, the completely flattened cells have become corneocytes without nuclei. Although these cells used to be considered dead, we have learned that they are still active and contain special organelles to help maintain stability. The compact layer, which is the lower, contains cells that are linked to one another. In the outer, sloughing layer, those links break down, and the cells gradually flake off.

This process of generation, maturation, and death of a cell takes about a month. As you age, cell renewal slows down and dead cells build up on the surface of the skin. This accumulation of dead cells makes skin appear dull.

Stratum Corneum Superstar: A New Assessment

In the past, the cornified layer was considered simply a dead layer of skin, a grave-yard of the inactive skeletons of keratinocytes that had completed their upward journey from the basal layer. It turns out that this layer is more than a lattice of dead keratin. The significance of this outermost layer had been overlooked for decades. Research-ers now know that the cornified layer has biologi-cal properties responsible for maintaining healthy skin. Rather than being inert, the cornified layer functions as a vital barrier that regulates water loss; prevents damage from external oxidants; limits infection through peptides that kill micro-organisms; has hormone receptors; launches an immune response to invading microbes, anti-gens, and allergens; and protects cells below from damaging ultraviolet light. The Lancer Method focuses on the cornified layer's role in stabilizing the skin and maintaining its structure. This is the secret at the heart of the Lancer Method, which uses the stratum corneum's messaging system to revive your skin and give it a youthful appearance.

The skin, like the rest of the body, actively maintains homeostasis—in other words, a sta-ble condition. With the dynamic and continual

Cell Turnover in the Epidermis

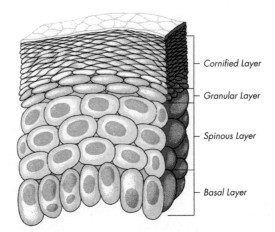

- Cornified Layer
- Granular Layer
- Spinous Layer
- Basal Layer

The epidermis normally never stops regenerating. Cells shaped like columns in the basal layer divide and push already formed cells into higher levels, where they flatten out. If you look at the shape of the cells, you will see that the closer they are to the skin's surface, the flatter they become.

process of cell formation in the epidermis, the skin maintains a constant number of cells. When dead cells flake off the cornified layer, they are replaced by the newly formed cells moving up from the granular layer. Homeostasis is regulated in part by the dermis. Since the epidermis does not have blood vessels, the outer layer of skin cannot initiate the production of new cells. Feedback loops and sensors in the cornified layer detect when the balance is off or when injury occurs. Hormones, growth factors, and cytokines do the signaling to the dermis, which then drives cell production. The cornified layer communicates with the dermis through these feedback loops to stimulate the skin's self-repair mechanism. The Lancer Method uses this natural process to speed up the production of new and healthy skin cells. The next chapter provides you with an in-depth explanation of how harnessing the skin's own healing process actually works.

Aging Changes in the Epidermis

- Even though the number of cell layers remains the same, the epidermis thins with age.
- There is some age-related loss of cellular and extracellular matrix.
- The pigment-containing cells, melanocytes, decrease in number but increase in size. This can produce the age spots that appear in sun-exposed areas of your skin.
- Aging skin can appear thinner and paler as a result of these changes.
- Cell turnover slows down. The process takes about twice as long when you are fifty as it did when you were twenty.
- Sun exposure and other environmental factors can strip the epidermis of protective anti-oxidants, resulting in oxidative stress.

HOW THE SKIN STAYS HYDRATED

The epidermis is responsible for keeping skin hydrated. Water is vital for the proper functioning and maintenance of the epidermis, and affects the outward appearance of healthy skin. If there is too much water, skin cells break down because of increased permeability. As you can imagine, too little hydration results in dryness. The epidermis contains the underlying mechanism that controls hydration, maintaining a balance between water retention and water loss. This complex process is still not fully understood by modern scientists, but we are able to use what knowledge we do have to our benefit.

Throughout the body, there are channels called aquaporins that facilitate the passage of water and small molecules. There are thirteen different types of aquaporins in your body. We are concerned with aquaporin 3 (AQP3), which are abundantly found in the membranes of the keratinocytes in the epidermis, primarily in the stratum basale. Moving toward the skin's surface, the number of these channels decreases with each layer of the epidermis. Water in the stratum corneum makes up only 10 to 15 percent of the content, compared with 75 percent in the underlying layers of the epidermis. This distribution allows living layers of the epidermis to remain well hydrated while water loss is minimized.

AQP3 transport water and glycerol into the cells of the epidermis. Glycerol acts as a humectant, a substance that promotes the retention of water. As the glycerol diffuses into the stratum corneum and underlying epidermis, it pulls water with it, hydrating the skin. This action provides elasticity and helps barrier repair in the epidermis. Glycerol also affects metabolism in the stratum corneum and the composition of lipids. With age or chronic sun exposure, the number of aquaporins decreases, which accounts for the dryness visible in aging or sun-damaged skin.

Skin Hydration through Aquaporin 3 Channel

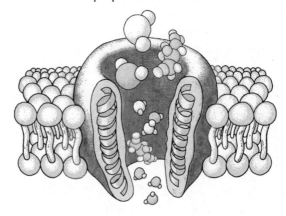

This closeup of an aquaporin 3 shows water and glycerol entering through a cell membrane.

The stratum corneum contains natural moisturizing factors, like urea, which contribute to maintaining the water level in the epidermis. Urea is a humectant that attracts water to the skin, particularly from the dermis. Most dermatologists focus on topical products to keep the skin hydrated. Glycerol and urea are ingredients in creams, lotions, shampoos, ointments, pastes, foams, and body washes. The Lancer Method not only prepares the skin to absorb moisturizing agents, but also increases the metabolism in the skin that helps to transport the active ingredients in topical treatments. As the Lancer Method speeds up production of new keratinocytes, the entire machine is upgraded. The aquaporins remain very active, and glycerol and urea continue to be produced, keeping the skin well hydrated.

Lifestyle Alone Is Not Enough—To Look Younger, You Need to Upgrade Your Skin Care

A very accomplished film executive was prompted to call my office because of an innocent observation from her five-year-old daughter. She had taken her daughter to the playground during the weekend and was talking to the group of mothers as they watched their children play there. On their way home, her daughter commented, "Mommy, you look older than the other mommies at the park."

The woman was stunned! In her late thirties, she had been proud of her slim figure and excellent physical condition. She thought she was doing a great job of having it all—a successful career, a good marriage, and an adorable little girl. Her daughter's remark made her take notice. She had been very health-oriented but realized that her approach to her looks had been non-cosmetic.

During our consultation, she made it clear that she did not want any major treatments, definitely no injections or fillers. What she wanted was to be more color-blended and radiant. She committed to trying the Lancer Method. After two or three days, she saw results. She looked fresher and less tired. She became a total convert. It took her child's innocent comment to inspire her to learn about beauty and skin care. The changes she saw with her own eyes proved to her that she needed more than a healthy lifestyle to slow down aging and to have younger-looking skin.

The Takeaway: An aging, poorly maintained face and a youthful body dominates the impression that you make and defines you. A luminous, even complexion makes you ageless.

You cannot be passive when it comes to taking care of your skin. Now that you have been introduced to the science behind the Lancer Method, it's time to act. The next chapter will explain what you have to do to tap into your skin's natural healing power to get the Lancer Glow. You will learn my simple technique—when and how to awaken your skin. Get ready to bring your skin back to life.

3

The Basic Lancer Anti-Aging Method

After I ask new patients, "What can I do for you?" I follow up with the question, "How do you care for your skin at home?" For years, we have had patients bring their skin care products with them for their first consultation. Usually, people fall into one of two camps. There are minimalists, men and women who tell me they use a facial cleanser or soap and put on a little moisturizer before bed. This approach will do nothing to preserve their skin and keep it looking young. On the other end of the spectrum are the product junkies who cannot resist the extreme claims and promises of the beauty trap sales machine. They are always trying the latest elixir promising to stop the clock, spending a fortune at cosmetics counters and drugstores. Their skin care regimens are elaborate and time consuming, but despite their efforts, nothing seems to give them the results they want.

I prescribe the Lancer Three-Step Method—Step one, Polish; Step two,

Cleanse; Step three, Nourish—to all of my patients, regardless of how sophisticated they are about cosmetics and how far they have gone with invasive procedures. The Lancer Method is simple and delivers on the promise of transforming your skin. You will achieve a vibrant glow and youthful fullness to your complexion for a moderate investment of time and money. The Lancer Method works so well, actually reversing the natural slowing of cellular function, that some people see improvements in as little as three to five days. You will rejuvenate your skin at home by naturally restoring a system that becomes damaged by time and lifestyle. The principle of the Lancer Method is to stimulate your skin to repair itself.

AN ANTI-AGING BREAKTHROUGH

The Lancer Method is so effective because it revolutionizes skin care. What is unique about my method is that it:

- Works for all skin types and ethnicities.
- Targets the epidermis, signaling a cascade of reparative action down to the dermis.
- Actually triggers skin cells to turn over more quickly, so skin repairs itself.
- Helps to address a range of skin issues and complaints, without the use of harsh chemicals or drying irritants.
- Increases oxygen transport throughout all skin layers.

ONE METHOD FOR ALL

One of the hallmarks of the Lancer Method is that it isn't based on the usual skin types—oily, dry, combination—as so many other programs are. While versions of the method have been optimized for sensitive or acne-prone skin, the action and the effect of these products are the same as the rest of the line. At Lancer Skincare, we treat problems based on inflammation. Inflammation is the body's self-protective response, triggered by the immune system to destroy harmful "invaders." Inflammation is at the root of all skin problems, from acne in a teenager to lines and wrinkles in a more mature face. Though acne and aging might seem unrelated, they are actually on the same spectrum of inflammation, causing breakouts in the teenager and precipitating collagen breakdown in the older person. From wrinkles to rosacea to hyperpigmentation, inflammation leads to complexion imperfections and aging. When properly controlled and induced, inflammation can also be harnessed to help repair the skin. This controlled inflammation, also known as controlled stimulation, is the crux of the Lancer Method. You are providing the environment for your skin to rejuvenate itself.

Another crucial aspect of the Lancer approach is the care we take in understanding a patient's genetic history—more specifically, his or her family's varied ethnicities. Globalization is a major aspect of the times in which we live, and as a result, complexion is no longer a telling sign of ancestry. Every shade of skin has a different reaction to injury, aging, and ingredients. As you will read in chapter 5, the Lancer Ethnicity Scale was developed in order to understand more fully how patients' genetic history may affect their reaction to a given treatment or procedure.

If you have acne, rosacea, or sensitive skin, you will use different skin care products for the Lancer Method, but the regimen remains the same. Read the specific chapter for your condition in part 2 before beginning the program.

THE LANCER METHOD TARGETS THE EPIDERMIS

The Lancer Method overturns traditional skin care by shifting the focus from the dermis to the epidermis. Most anti-aging skin care products and regimens available today focus on the dermis. One reason many dermis-focused skin care systems are not effective is that the ingredients, no matter how exotic, are unable to advance change as effectively as the skin's intrinsic system does. Even if those ingredients have therapeutic powers, they often do not reach the skin they are trying to treat. All those expensive ingredients in anti-aging creams and serums will not be able to do the work of restoring and repairing the skin if they cannot reach the dermis. The skin must be stimulated to repair itself!

TO LOOK YOUNGER, YOUR SKIN NEEDS TO BE EXFOLIATED EVERY DAY

With the Lancer Method, you will start by exfoliating or polishing the epidermis, the skin's top layer, to lay the foundation for transforming your complexion. Dermatologists tend to pay cursory attention to exfoliation, treating it as an adjunct to cleansing. Most experts recommend a gentle cleanse, followed by a toner to remove residue, then the application of a super-nutrient skin cream, and finally sunblock. I view exfoliation—or as I like to call it, polishing—as the key to perking up your skin cells, which get sluggish as you age. Polishing is a crucial step to restarting the repairing activity of your skin cells.

What, No Toner?

Most skin care regimens include a toner step, but not everyone needs one. Toners are primarily formulated to return the skin to its natural pH level. The pH is the balance between acidity and alkalinity in your body. The skin on the face is at its healthiest when it is slightly acidic. Acid prohibits bacterial growth that can contribute to acne and helps maintain the skin's barrier function, keeping moisture in and harmful substances out. Alkaline skin is more prone to lines, wrinkles, and sun damage.

All that would seem to make toner a must, but if you have relatively normal skin, exfoliate regularly, and use a cleanser that does not strip your skin of its natural moisture, you should be able to maintain a healthy pH level. Lifestyle changes will do the rest.

A NEW ORDER

The first step of the Lancer Method is polishing, followed by cleansing, and then nourishing. This change in the traditional order of skin care allows for a deeper cleanse, more efficient delivery of active ingredients, and more robust cell renewal. Let me explain in construction terms. Say you want to replace a tile floor. If your epidermis is the floor, then exfoliation is the gentle lifting process that breaks up the old, worn-out tiles. Next you have to scoop up and sweep away the debris, the cleanse step in the Lancer Method that washes away exfoliant, excess oil, and dirt. Finally, new, fresh tiles have to be laid, and that is accomplished in the Lancer Method by the nourish step, which stimulates rapid self-repair of the skin.

THE LANCER METHOD USES CONTROLLED INFLAMMATION TO REFRESH YOUR SKIN

Exfoliation creates "controlled injury." Gentle exfoliation sends a message to the dermis that repair should begin and fresh cells are needed, expediting the turnover of cells in your epidermis. When you are young, facial cell renewal occurs at a rapid pace, which is one of the reasons young skin looks so vibrant and dewy. As you age, the process slows down. The controlled injury achieved by exfoliating turns back the clock by reenergizing the repair process, giving skin a younger, fresher look.

Controlled, repetitive, mechanical stimulation reaches deeper than the epidermis to improve the appearance of your skin. Controlled stimulation of the epidermis signals a cascade of responses in your body. A complex repair process kicks in as if you had a true injury. When the stratum corneum barrier is "damaged," pathways of inflammation are activated by the cytokines produced by the immune system, growth factors, and other hormones. Epidermal growth factors are proteins that regulate cellular growth and activity. These messengers produce an immune response to the injury—or perceived injury—activated to repair the wound evenly and quickly. Epidermal growth factor supports cell renewal by increasing the production of proteins, fibroblasts, collagen, and blood vessels, as well as boosting circulation—all of which keep your skin looking young. Ultraviolet light slows down the production of epidermal growth factor, which directly affects your skin's ability to repair itself. This is one of the main reasons unprotected exposure to sunlight ages your skin prematurely.

When you exfoliate, you are signaling controlled inflammation in the skin. The injury your skin experiences is like muscle aches after a hard workout. *No pain, no gain*, as my trainer likes to remind me. You need controlled injury or inflammation to produce the desired result—younger, dewy skin. The inflammation you have created by exfoliating causes the arterial capillaries to dilate. These blood vessels contain oxygenated blood, which is red and carries more oxygen to the skin. You can see this in the slight pink flush of your skin after polishing. Increased oxygen metabolism in the dermis sets in motion cellular activities that decrease the external signs of aging. When blood vessels stretch, the inside of the vessels release hormone signals that stimulate the fibroblasts. The inflamed cells swell and are distorted. This revs up the engine inside the fibroblasts, preparing them to produce collagen. The process is like a dormant factory going into production. This controlled inflammation creates powerful anti-aging action in the skin.

Exfoliation ultimately stimulates the body's mechanism for rebuilding collagen, the key to restoring your skin. The Lancer Method relies upon the anatomy of the skin to oxygenate itself and to build up growth factor, collagen, glycerol, hyaluronic acid, and other youth-promoting elements that otherwise diminish with age.

THE PRODUCT JUNGLE

Just walk into the skin care aisle of the local drugstore or the first floor of a department store or leaf through a fashion magazine. The number of beautifully packaged products making big promises is daunting. Confronting the overwhelming selection of skin care products is like being lost in an overgrown jungle full of exotic plants, vines, and flowers, and you do not know the way out or where danger might be lurking. The choices out there are dizzying. There are countless products claiming transformative powers, and some of them are fine. How do you begin to pick the best from the overwhelming number of choices—those cleansers, creams, serums, and lotions that will be effective? I will guide you through the overabundance of products and help you make the right choices.

This chapter contains my recommendations for the highest-quality products, from my own Lancer Skincare products to other luxury brands, from moderately priced products to very affordable ones. Knowing what works cuts through the confusion the beauty trap creates. Cosmetics companies are always pushing new ingredients that they claim are miraculous. I can tell you that they are not. Since most product labels read like a foreign language, I will provide you with the active ingredients to look for and those to avoid.

Keep Your Skin Care Products Effective

I recommend that you keep your skin care products in the refrigerator to extend their life. You have invested in high-quality products. You do not want them to turn, spoil, or become contaminated. Throw away products that have been around too long and have turned brown. The color change in the product indicates that it has oxidized and lost potency. Many of my patients use small "six-pack" refrigerators that they keep in the bathroom.

EXPAND THE TREATMENT TERRITORY

If you want to continue wearing low-cut necklines and avoid having to rely on turtlenecks and scarves to hide your neck, you have to take care of the delicate skin below your jawline, namely your neck and décolletage. Too many people focus on their faces and ignore those vulnerable areas that are exposed to just as many damaging UV rays as the face. The fact is, your neck and chest need as much attention as your face, if not more. Both areas tend to show signs of aging before facial skin. The skin of the neck and décolletage is thinner and does not have as much collagen to begin with. There are fewer oil glands in these areas as well. The skin of the chest area is more sensitive than other parts of the body, has less elasticity, and has little fat tissue to act as a cushion. These physical characteristics explain why the neck becomes lined and saggy and the skin surrounding the cleavage can develop lines, wrinkles, blotches, redness, and hyperpigmentation.

With the Lancer Method, you take care of your skin "from the dinner table up"—your face, neck, chest, shoulders, and upper back—twice a day. We will get to the hands and arms later. You should apply the three-step method from your hairline to the sun-shielded area of your chest, including your shoulders and your back. You never know when you are going to wear a strapless dress or one that is cut low in back. Treat these areas the same way as your face, because you want the skin of your face, neck, and chest to match. A turkey neck and crepey décolletage will age you no matter how good your face looks. Do not forget your arms and hands, particularly if you drive a lot. UV rays can do damage through your windshield.

MAKEUP REMOVAL

If you wear makeup, you will have to remove all cosmetics before you polish at night. There is no reason to buy makeup remover. Invest the money you save in higher-quality products. The aestheticians at Lancer Skincare use olive oil or grape seed oil to remove makeup. If olive oil feels too heavy for your skin, grape seed oil is much lighter. Keep a travel-size plastic bottle filled with oil with your skin care products. Squirt a quarter-size amount of oil onto the palm of your hand and apply with your fingertips to your face, to your neck, and as far as your makeup goes. Gently wipe off your makeup with a soft tissue. Rinse your face and neck with warm water and leave your skin damp, not wet. Now you are ready to polish.

Another option is to use your cleanser to remove your makeup, then polish and cleanse again. If your cleanser can get rid of sebum and pollution, it should be able to remove your makeup, even mascara. Just remember to follow the three steps after you remove your makeup.

THE LANCER METHOD: POLISH, CLEANSE, NOURISH

The Lancer Method changes the order of your skin care routine. With most skin regimens, you cleanse and then moisturize. As you now know, polishing is the important first step in the regimen, followed by cleansing, then nourishing. You will be polishing only once a day—that is all you need to stimulate your skin. I suggest that you exfoliate at night before you go to bed. Your skin repairs itself more efficiently while you sleep. During your sleeping hours, other processes in your body slow down. With fewer demands, your body can direct more energy to healing and restoring your skin.

If you exfoliate at night, you skip that step in the morning, but the number of steps remains at three. You will replace the polish step by adding protection at the end of your morning routine. Sunscreen should not be reserved for the beach. Applying sunscreen to your face, neck, chest, hands, and lower arms—and all areas of your body exposed to the sun as you go through the day—is a crucial defense against skin aging. Daily protection is so important that I have built it into my simple skin care routine. You should keep your sunscreen with your skin care products and carry some with you during the day so that you can reapply.

THE BASIC LANCER ANTI-AGING METHOD

My skin care routine is simple and will not take you more than ten minutes a day. That small time investment will yield big results. Many people see improvements in their skin in a matter of days.

Unless you have cornrows, dreadlocks, or helmet head, you would not go through a day without brushing or combing your hair! You do not give a thought to running a comb through your hair. Skin hygiene is equally important to your appearance over the long term. Make it automatic, habitual—an essential part of your grooming. Incorporating this three-step morning and evening routine into your day is not challenging. When you see what a difference the Lancer Method makes, taking care of your skin will become a pleasure.

To restore your skin's radiance, refine your pores, correct unevenness in your skin tone, lift your complexion, and reduce the signs of aging, this is all you have to do:

A.M.
1. Cleanse
2. Nourish
3. Protect

P.M.
1. Polish
2. Cleanse
3. Nourish

That is it. This is all you have to do to treat your skin on a daily basis. Even the busiest person can manage this. You might find it hard to believe that such a simple program delivers the promised results. Try it. You will become a convert to the Lancer Method.

Step 1: Polish

Polishing is a skin energizer, and the key to the Lancer Method. I prefer to use the word *polish* over *exfoliate*, because it provides a good visual image of how removing dead skin cells is like taking the tarnish off silver. Polishing allows fresh, radiant skin to shine through. The number one benefit of this step is that skin instantly feels smoother and silkier. Of course, polishing goes deeper than that. This step changes the physiology of your skin to make it act younger. The restoration of your skin's radiance is a sign of all the work going on below to support cell renewal and to increase collagen production in your dermis.

You can exfoliate your skin in two different ways: mechanically and chemically. Mechanical polishers could be anything from a loofah or rough washcloth to a scrub with tiny grains or crystals that rub off dead cells. Chemical polishers are made of enzyme-based ingredients from plants like papaya and pineapple that dissolve dead cells. A combination of both tiny scrubbers and enzymes works best. Loofahs and washcloths do not do the job as well. Mechanical polishers can harbor bacteria unless you launder them after every use.

The Anti-Aging Benefits of Polishing

When you exfoliate, you:

- Remove dead skin cells that make your skin look dull and flaky.
- Give your skin a rosy glow by increasing oxygenation.
- Stimulate the production of epidermal growth factor.
- Accelerate cell turnover, which slows as you age, for fresher-looking skin.
- Plump up your skin by creating controlled inflammation that leads to the production of collagen.
- Allow nourishing skin care products to penetrate better by removing the surface layer of dead cells, which otherwise limits how much lotion penetrates.
- Further improve the moisture balance of your skin by stimulating natural moisturizing factors.

Polishing Technique

The secret to polishing is to be gentle. You are not trying to rub your skin raw. Let the product do the work. The best place to exfoliate is in the shower, because you will be exfoliating your face, neck, chest, shoulders, and the top of your back.

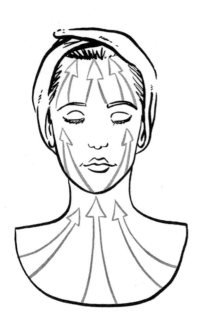

Rinsing off is much easier in the shower. If you do not shower at night, you should still polish at the end of your day. Just rinse off at the sink. Polishing should take sixty to ninety seconds. You might want to set a timer the first few times so that you know what a minute to a minute and a half feels like.

You may need to ease into a polishing routine. If you have never exfoliated the skin of your face or haven't done so for a long time, your skin may react by getting red and dry. Do not be alarmed if this happens, because it's a sign that the exfoliation is working. If your skin gets dry and flaky, polish every other day until your skin adjusts.

When exfoliating, cleansing, or nourishing, always work upward, against gravity. Start with your jawline and work to your hairline. Then work up from where the lighter skin begins on your chest, up your neck, to your jawline. Do not forget the sides of your neck and your upper back.

Just follow these directions every night:

- Dampen the skin on your face, neck, and chest with warm water.
- Place a small amount of polish—about the size of a pea—on your fingertips. Make sure to use enough polish, with repeat portions when necessary. Ten pea-size droplets may be needed just for the face!
- Beginning at your chin, gently massage your skin in a circular motion. Pay special attention to your chin, nose, and forehead, where blackheads and whiteheads tend to develop.
- If you have lines on the sides of your lips, push out the folds with your tongue and work that skin.
- Push your nose aside with one hand and gently polish the crease at the outer side of your nostril. Repeat on the other side.
- Do not forget your lips.
- Do not polish the sensitive skin around your eyes.

- When you have finished your face, start at your bra line or where your skin is white and work up your chest, neck, and jawline with the same circular motion. Use more polish if necessary. Do not forget the sides of the neck.
- Polish your shoulders and your upper back as well.
- Rinse with lukewarm water. A polish film will remain, which is part of the interlocking chemistry.

You have now set in motion a process of rejuvenation at the cellular level.

What to Look for in a Polisher

I prefer a polisher that uses a combination of mechanical, natural, and synthetic exfoliants. The mechanical scrubbers are often sea minerals, and chemical polishers may be fruit extracts. Most products are made with either one or the other type of exfoliant. If faced with a choice, go for the mechanical exfoliants, preferably one made with sea minerals. If there is a sample, feel the polisher before you buy. The scrubbers should be superfine. The product should not feel like sandpaper and should have enough emollient to feel comfortable on your skin. That is the mark of high-quality chemistry. Large mechanical exfoliants can abrade the skin, causing irritation.

If you prefer to use the type of polisher that dissolves dead cells, look for one with natural exfoliating enzymes. Lancer Skincare uses natural phytocompounds, which are plant-based enzymes. Fruit-based enzymes are less irritating and have more predictable reactions with a wide range of skin types. Since exfoliation is central to beautiful skin, a very high-quality polisher is worth splurging on.

Recommended Exfoliators

Luxury:
Lancer Skincare The Method: Polish
Chanel Gommage Microperlé Éclat
AmorePacific Bio-Enzyme Refining
    Complex Self-Activating Skin
    Polisher
Kanebo Sensai Silky Purifying
    Cleansing Gel with Scrub
La Mer The Refining Facial

Moderate:
Dermalogica Multivitamin Thermafoliant

Elizabeth Arden Ceramide Plump
    Perfect Gentle Line Smoothing
    Exfoliator

Affordable:
RoC Daily Resurfacing Disks
L'Oréal Paris Go 360° Clean Deep
    Exfoliating Scrub

Avoid walnut shell or almond shell powder. These are sharp, uneven particles that are too harsh for a facial exfoliator.

Step 2: Cleanse

If you think of exfoliating as going into a mine and blowing up the rocks surrounding the gems, cleansing is moving in a cart to carry all the debris away. Cleansing helps you to get rid of everything that you have loosened up by exfoliating. Many cleansers contain some chemical exfoliating ingredients. If you use such a cleanser, you will extend the polishing process, further refining the stratum corneum and prepping the skin for nourishment. For most people, I am an advocate of using a cleanser with exfoliating ingredients.

When you cleanse, you want to remove any makeup and sunscreen that remain, plus dirt and bacteria. You do not want to strip your skin completely, leaving it dry and irritated. Though cleansing helps to dissolve sebum and other greasy substances that get trapped in the pores, you still need to keep the skin's natural oils intact. It is a balancing act, but a good cleanser will help you find a happy medium. One surprisingly good option is simple baby shampoo, a gentle but thorough cleanser you can use on your face and body.

The Anti-Aging Benefits of Cleansing

- Gentle removal of debris, makeup, perspiration, dirt, oil, and bacteria that can dull the skin.
- Continuing the exfoliating process with the right facial cleanser.
- Eliminating blackheads.
- Keeping your pores from getting clogged so that the skin can breathe.
- Refining enlarged pores.
- Preparing the skin to receive the active ingredients in the nourishing step.
- The cleanser's chemistry should interlock with the polishing and nourishing products for maximum benefit.

What to Look for in a Cleanser

Your goal is to find a cleanser that is non-irritating, non-inflammatory, and soothing, but still thoroughly cleans your skin. Stay away from heavily scented cleansers. After washing your face, your skin should feel free of any filminess, but not so squeaky-clean that your face feels taut or itchy. Washing with soap will make your skin feel that way. Soap strips the skin of natural oils and can leave a residue at the same time. To clean your face gently, it is worth getting a facial cleanser specifically formulated to clean deeply without stripping the skin. A good cleanser can be used on your entire face, including eyelids, neck, and chest. If you usually use a bar of soap or a spritz of liquid soap to cleanse, it's time to change that habit if you want your skin to look younger.

I do recommend using an exfoliating cleanser. Look for salicylic acid or alpha hydroxy acids (AHA) on the label. Even though cleanser remains on your face for a short time, these ingredients will help to remove dead cells and give a boost to the cell renewal process.

To avoid creating a product that is overly drying, many cosmetics companies add substances that promote water retention, called humectants, and other moisture-gathering compounds to their formulas. The problem is that these cleansers often leave a film on the skin. For anti-aging purposes you should choose a stronger cleanser without the moisturizing add-ins.

Most cosmetic cleansers employ synthetic cleansers called syndets that are pH-neutral and do not leave a film on the skin. Two that you will commonly see are sodium cocoyl isethionate, derived from coconuts; and sodium palmitate, from palm trees. The Lancer Method uses sodium PCA to adjust the pH of the skin to prepare it for nourishment, and to bind water to the skin's surface. Our formula also uses aloe vera glycosides, which accelerate cell renewal. A rice protein and an amino acid compound regulate water channeling through the aquaporin on a cellular level, ensuring that skin is smooth, hydrated, and soothed.

If possible, try the product before you buy a cleanser. Rub a little on the soft skin on the inside of your arm. If the cleanser does not cause redness or irritation, the product will most likely be fine for your face, neck, and chest.

Cleansing Technique

It should take you only sixty seconds to cleanse your face. No matter how tired you are, remember that going to bed with clean, freshly nourished skin will allow your skin to regenerate while you sleep. Maintenance is the key to younger-looking skin. You should use the same technique as you do for the polish step:

- At night, your skin will already be damp from having just been polished. In the morning, wet your skin a bit before cleansing.
- Place a pea-size drop of cleanser on your fingertips and work it onto your face first from the jawline up. Starting just below your jawline and moving upward, massage your face, including your eye area.
- Add more cleanser if needed.

- Rinse well with tepid water and pat dry.
- Working up from your bra line, repeat for your chest, shoulders, upper back, and neck.

The skin is an organ of absorption. Your face is exposed to many harmful pollutants, chemicals, and bacteria, which are absorbed through the skin and cause uncontrolled inflammation. Keeping your skin meticulously clean will reduce the toxic load in your body, and preventing the buildup of toxins is a very effective anti-aging strategy.

Proper cleansing prepares your skin to absorb the nutrients you will apply in the next step.

Recommendations for Facial Cleansers

Using a cleanser created specifically for the face will help to preserve and restore your skin. I prefer cleansers that contain some mild exfoliants to extend the effects of the polish step. These cleansers will neither dry your skin nor leave a residue.

Luxury:
Lancer Skincare The Method: Cleanse
Chanel Sublimage Essential Comfort Cleanser
AmorePacific Treatment Cleansing Oil Face & Eyes
Le Métier de Beauté Skin Renewal Cleanser

Kanebo Sensai Silky Purifying Cleansing Milk

Moderate:
Dermalogica Dermal Clay Cleanser
Elizabeth Arden Ceramide Purifying Cream Cleanser
Kiehl's Clearly Corrective Purifying Foaming Cleanser
Estée Lauder Perfectly Clean Foam Cleanser/Purifying Mask

Affordable:
RoC MAX Resurfacing Facial Cleanser
L'Oréal Paris Youth Code Youth Regenerating Skincare Foaming Gel Cleanser

---

Step 3: Nourish

This step gives new meaning to the phrase *feeding your face*. When you use a well-formulated product, you are delivering important nutrients your skin needs to repair and protect itself from the aging process. Though most nourishing products help the skin retain moisture, their main role is to deliver anti-oxidants, vitamins, and other anti-aging ingredients to the stratum corneum and the layers below.

In addition, Lancer Skincare Nourish contains firming and anti-inflammatory ingredients. A good nourisher will quench and control inflammation.

When you open up the doors of the skin, which you do by polishing and cleansing, you allow active ingredients to penetrate, provided that the product is well formulated. Nourishers also seal the skin, locking in the ingredients that help heal the controlled injury, giving the skin the nutrients it needs to rebuild itself.

What You Want in a Nourisher

Nourishers come in many forms, including lotion, cream, and serum formulations, and they are called by many names. They may be labeled as "reparative lotions," "anti-aging creams," or "anti-wrinkle treatments." The single most important ingredient of the nourishing step is anti-oxidants. There are many anti-oxidants used in skin care products, and one is not necessarily better than the next. The various anti-oxidants use different metabolic pathways to protect the skin. Vitamin C and vitamin E are two anti-oxidants commonly found in nourishing products. Provided they are present in adequate amounts and in stable forms, these vitamins are very effective.

Vitamin C helps stop free radicals created by sun exposure from doing damage and may even provide a barrier to the sun's rays. Vitamin C protects collagen and stimulates the fibroblasts to produce more. Look for vitamin C in the form of L-ascorbic acid, which offers the best anti-aging results.

Vitamin E is another efficient free radical scavenger, fighting inflammation. It also functions to keep the skin moisturized. Vitamin E is a preservative as well, used to keep cosmetics from spoiling. It usually appears on the ingredients listing as alpha-tocopherol. If you see it on the list, make sure vitamin E is close to the top. Otherwise, the anti-oxidant might be in the product as a preservative. There may not be an adequate amount to make your skin younger.

A good nourishing product may include peptides and pentapeptides. The peptide group of amino acids, the building blocks of protein, has a range of anti-aging effects. When collagen breaks down, it forms peptides; the peptides signal the skin to make new collagen. Topical peptides have been shown to do the same.

Finally, select a nourisher that feels good on your skin. I recommend avoiding heavily scented creams and serums, because the fragrances can cause your skin to react. If your nourisher feels luxurious and your skin feels soft when you put it on, you will look forward to using it rather than conveniently "forgetting" this step. When you take care of your skin, you should feel pampered. As the benefits begin to show, the Lancer Method will be an intrinsic part of your grooming routine that you would not dream of skipping.

Nourishing Technique

At night, nourishing your skin is the last step. In the morning, nourishing is followed by protecting your skin. In either case, you have prepared your skin to receive anti-aging ingredients that will help to preserve or restore its firmness and visibly diminish the appearance of lines and wrinkles. You will use the nourishing cream, lotion, or serum on the same area of skin you treated in the previous steps.

- Place a pea-size drop of nourishing cream, lotion, or serum on your fingertips.
- Working from the jawline to the hairline, apply your nourishing product gently in circular strokes.
- Most nourishers can be applied to the delicate skin around the eye.
- Add more nourisher if needed.
- Repeat the process from your bra line or where the skin is lighter on your chest up to the jawline.
- Be certain to do the sides of your neck and upper back.

Recommendations for Moisturizers

Luxury:
Lancer Skincare The Method: Nourish
Chanel Sublimage La Crème
AmorePacific Time Response Renewal Creme
La Prairie Anti-Aging Day Cream SPF 30
Kanebo Sensai Silk Emulsion (Moist)

Moderate:
Dermalogica Dynamic Skin Recovery SPF 30

Kiehl's Powerful Wrinkle Reducing Cream
Estée Lauder DayWear Oil-Free

Affordable:
RoC Deep Wrinkle Daily Moisturizer with SPF
Jergens Age Defying Multi-Vitamin Moisturizer
L'Oréal Paris Revitalift Anti-Wrinkle & Firming Day Cream SPF 18

Step 3 Morning Routine: Protect

Sun exposure accelerates skin aging—it is as simple as that. You can use the best of serums, creams, and lotions, but they cannot do their job if you continue to expose your skin to the sun without protection. You are wasting your time and money. The damaging effects of UV rays will counteract the healing action of the peptides, anti-oxidants, and other ingredients, and sun damage will prevail. Protection from UV rays must be part of your daily routine.

The degree of skin aging that results from UV rays is determined by your skin pigmentation and total lifetime sun exposure. The pigment melanin provides some protection against the sun. People with darker complexions have more melanin than those with fair skin, which is why it takes them longer to burn. The skin protects itself from the damaging effects of the sun by increasing production of the dark brown pigment melanin—in other words, tanning. Though fair-skinned people show more aging skin changes earlier than people with darker, more heavily pigmented skin, even the darkest skin is damaged by the sun. With dark skin, melanocytes can become overactive, producing a blotchy, mottled complexion. All skin is susceptible to sun-induced wrinkles. No one is exempt—everyone must use sunscreen, even if burning is not an issue. The good news is that the moment you start to protect your skin, you will put the brakes on additional damage and start to reverse what you have already accumulated.

Beyond aging, skin cancer is a real consideration. Figures from the Skin Cancer Foundation are startling:

- One in five Americans will develop skin cancer in his or her lifetime.
- One in three cancers diagnosed in the United States is skin cancer.
- Eighty percent of skin cancers occur on the head, neck, and hands, which are most exposed to the sun.
- The incidence of people under thirty developing melanoma is increasing faster than any other demographic group, soaring by 50 percent in young women since 1980.

Not all skin cancers are deadly, but dealing with them might require surgical removal, which is costly and can result in scarring. Sun exposure increases the risk of the most serious form of skin cancer, melanoma. The Skin Cancer Foundation has announced that melanoma rates are rising. Melanoma does have a good survival rate if you catch it early, but that rate falls to 15 percent if the cancer advances. Using sunscreen daily will help protect you from developing skin cancer.

Beware Mixing Some Medicines and Chemical Ingredients with the Sun

Here is another reason to use sunscreen every day. In reaction to UV rays, certain chemicals and drugs can make your skin more sensitive to the sun, causing inflammation in the form of sunburn, an eczema-like reaction, or hives. This interaction is known as photosensitivity. The reaction may be an allergic reaction or a direct toxic effect. With a photo-allergic reaction, UV exposure changes the structure of the drug so that the immune system sees the drug as an invader or antigen. The immune system initiates an allergic response that causes inflammation of the skin in the sun-exposed areas. A photo-allergic response resembles eczema, and the reaction is long lasting. In a photo-toxic reaction, the drug is activated by sun exposure and causes skin damage. The reaction looks like a bad sunburn.

If you are taking any of the drugs or using products with photosensitive ingredients from the following list, stay out of the sun or be very careful of sun exposure.

Toxic Effect
- Non-steroidal anti-inflammatory drugs (NSAIDs), better known as ibuprofen and aspirin
- Antibiotics
- Diuretics
- Anti-depressants
- Anti-anxiety medications
- Anti-psychotics
- Coal tar derivatives
- Retinoids and medications containing retinoic acid
- Oral medications used for diabetes
- Anti-fungals
- Anti-malarial drugs
- Chemotherapy agents

Allergic Reactions
- Fragrances found in personal grooming items and cosmetics
- Sunscreens with PABA
- Industrial cleaners that contain salicylanilide

Sunscreen that contains zinc or titanium can prevent photosensitivity.

THERE IS NO SUCH THING AS ALL-DAY PROTECTION

There is a broad array of sun protection products currently on the market, and that is a good thing. But with all these new products come hype and confusion, and when it comes to protecting your skin, you need the facts. Do not be fooled by the claim that a sunscreen will give you "all day protection." To start, *SPF* stands for "sun protection factor" and refers to how long you can stay out in the sun without burning. This number is calculated by comparing the time needed for a person to burn unprotected with how long it takes for that person to burn wearing sunscreen.

SPF sunscreens help to protect the skin from short-wave UVB rays, not long-wave UVA rays. It is important to use full-spectrum sunscreen that will protect your skin from both long-wave UVAs and short-wave UVBs. As you will recall, UVBs are the rays that cause sunburn, and UVAs are those that cause sun damage.

SPF is meant to indicate the maximum sun exposure time the sunscreen will allow without burning. So if you typically burn in 10 minutes without protection, wearing an SPF of 15, you would theoretically be able to stay in the sun for 150 minutes without burning. The SPF number is not an exact measure by any means. The effectiveness of sunscreen depends on your skin tone, how much sunscreen you apply, the time of day you are exposed to the sun's rays, and your activities.

It might be logical to think that an SPF of 30 is twice as good as an SPF of 15, but that is not how it works. An SPF 15 product blocks about 94 percent of UVB

Recommended Sunscreens

I am recommending some products that combine sunscreen with a moisturizer.

Luxury:

Lancer Skincare Sheer Fluid Sun Shield SPF 30

Chanel UV Essentiel SPF 30

AmorePacific Natural Protector SPF 30/PA+++

La Prairie Advanced Marine Biology Day Cream SPF 20

Erno Laszlo Firmarine Moisturizer SPF 30

Jurlique Sun Lotion SPF 30+

Aesop Sage & Zinc Facial Hydrating Cream SPF 15

Moderate:

Dermalogica Daily Defense Block SPF 15

Elizabeth Arden Ceramide Premiere Activation Cream SPF 30

Estée Lauder DayWear Advanced Multi-Protection Anti-Oxidant & UV Defense SPF 50

Clarins Bright Plus HP Brightening Hydrating Day Lotion SPF 20

Clarins Sun Control Stick For Sun-Sensitive Areas SPF 30

Clinique City Block Sheer Oil-Free Daily Face Protector Broad Spectrum SPF 25

Affordable:

Neutrogena Clear Face Liquid-Lotion Sunscreen Broad Spectrum SPF 30

La Roche-Posay Anthelios 45 Ultra Light Fluid for Face

L'Oréal Paris Sublime Sun Advanced Sunscreen Liquid Silk Lotion SPF 30

Aveeno Positively Radiant Daily Moisturizer Broad Spectrum SPF 30

Cetaphil Daily Facial Moisturizer With Sunscreen Broad Spectrum SPF 15

rays, SPF 30 blocks 97 percent, and an SPF 45 product blocks 98 percent. Sunscreens with higher SPF ratings block slightly more UVB rays, but none offer 100 percent protection. SPFs used to top out at 30, but the race is on among sunscreen makers to create stratospheric SPFs. Do not let extremely high SPF numbers lull you into a false sense of security. The difference between an SPF 100 and an SPF 30 is marginal. When it comes to preventing signs of aging, you have to be hypervigilant about protecting your skin from the sun.

MAKE A COMMITMENT

The ability to look younger is in your own hands. The Lancer Method is state-of-the-art skin hygiene that you can practice at home. You have to commit to doing the routine twice a day no matter what. The Lancer Method does not demand a lot of your time: Just five to ten minutes a day is all that it takes to awaken your skin. To see improvement, you have to be consistent. I can always tell whether my patients are following the program. The effects of the Lancer Method are that noticeable. Without dedication to your skin routine, the dead cells you remove through the polish and cleanse steps will accumulate again, and cell renewal will slow considerably. Skin is alive, which is why you can change and improve it. If you stop taking care of your skin, it will revert to its previous state.

Renegade Regrets

I stayed in the office until midnight one Friday night to take care of an influential television producer and personality in his mid-forties. His assistant claimed he was desperately in need of help. He was driven straight from the airport. A patient for more than five years, he was a beautifully maintained racehorse.

He arrived at the office red-faced and so puffy his eyes were almost shut. His quest for constant maintenance had gotten him into trouble. Knowing he had gone too far, he came straight to Lancer Skincare. He encounters so many makeup artists and other experts on a regular basis that he is constantly at the mercy of people suggesting new things or offering him complimentary products and treatments in the hope of getting an endorsement. This time he had succumbed to the offer of a new, revitalizing treatment. He paid the price for his weak moment with a fried face. Four hours of treatments later, he left looking and feeling better. He resolved not to leave his anti-aging wingman again.

The Takeaway: When you find a skin care program that works, do not be tempted by novelties. You can always tweak your program to keep it interesting.

You now know how to perform "Lancer Magic." To transform your skin, the steps you have learned need to become second nature to you. Whether you are in a great rush in the morning or have been out late and just want to fall into bed, doing the three steps has to become automatic. You would not go out in the morning without brushing your teeth. Similarly, the Lancer Method has to be part of your regular routine. Incorporating the three steps into your life twice a day will be easy, especially when you see the results.

When I developed my theory of do-it-yourself controlled stimulation to make positive changes in the skin, I was confident that the Lancer Method would work. I was less confident that the available products could trigger the self-healing actions necessary to stimulate the skin to behave younger. I developed my own products for Lancer Skincare with the idea that skin care products could do more. I operated on the premise that if I took ingredients proven to have therapeutic value, used them in the right proportions, sequenced them appropriately, and wrapped it all up into formulations so sensuous that people would enjoy using them, the combination of the Lancer Method and the products could dramatically improve my patients' skin. I am not shy about saying that I know my own products are among the highest quality you can get, but my method will work with other products available on the market as well. Of course, you can also use other skin care products and still obtain good results with the Lancer Method if you follow the guidelines in this chapter. I want everyone to benefit from the Lancer Method regardless of budget. That is why I recommend acceptable products you can find in your local drugstores, price clubs, and department stores.

Ingredients: The Big Picture

The list that follows is a quick overview of desirable ingredients and those to avoid in your skin care products.

Active Ingredients to Look For

Hyaluronic acid: This component of connective tissues cushions and lubricates. Hyaluronic acid is found abundantly in your skin, but decreases with age. Smoking and diet lower levels as well. It is used topically in conjunction with vitamin C to treat wrinkled skin.

Peptides: These short snippets of linked amino acids reduce the appearance of wrinkles and fine lines. They stimulate collagen production.

Vitamins A, C, and E: These antioxidants prevent free radical damage and combat oxidation.

Bioactive phytocompounds: Phytocompounds are exciting new

(continued)

ingredients that have been isolated from natural plant sources. Not only are they natural, but many are very effective. For example, some of the best products contain natural fruit enzymes, moisturizing ingredients from sea algae and aloe vera, grape polyphenol, lilac stem cells, skin lighteners from licorice root, and anti-inflammatory agents from gingerroot. Natural tea tree oil, chamomile oil, and marula oil are also proven to be quite effective.

Possible Ingredients to Avoid

DEA (diethanolamine) and TEA (triethanolamine): These additives are used to adjust the pH in products and do double duty as emulsifiers. They can combine with nitrates to form carcinogens that cause liver and kidney damage.

Triclosan: An anti-bacterial chemical that may disrupt your hormones.

Petrolatum and petroleum distillates: Processed crude oil is used as an anti-foaming agent. Crude oil is toxic in any form.

DMDM hydantoin: This preservative can interact with other chemicals and release formaldehyde, a neurotoxin and carcinogen.

Dibutyl phthalate: The widely used fragrance enhancer disrupts hormones and interferes with reproduction.

Coal tar dye: This ingredient is made from petroleum and used to treat psoriasis and dandruff. It appears on labels as "FD&C" and "D&C."

BHT (butylated hydroxytoluene): Used as a preservative and anti-oxidant, BHT—which slows down the rate of color change in products—has been banned in other countries. It's a hormone disruptor that causes metabolic stress.

Parabens: This family of preservatives has anti-bacterial properties. It mimics estrogen and has been linked to breast cancer.

Benzoyl peroxide: An anti-acne agent, this ingredient can irritate the skin, eyes, and lungs.

Artificial dyes: Some artificial colors, like Blue 1 and Green 3, are carcinogenic. They are labeled "FD&C" or "D&C."

PABA: Once a common sunscreen ingredient, PABA can cause photosensitivity and has carcinogenic potential.

Benzene: This solvent, found in crude oil, gasoline, and cigarette smoke, is used in nail polish. It can be toxic and can irritate the skin, eyes, and lungs. It is a known carcinogen.

Anything to which you have a known sensitivity.

As the skin of your face, neck, décolletage, and shoulders improves, chances are you will start to notice signs of aging on the rest of your body. The Lancer Anti-Aging Method for Body will help you restore your skin from head to toe.

4

The Lancer Anti-Aging Method for Body

People spend so much money and time on their appearance from chin to hairline and do very little for the rest of their bodies. In the previous chapter, you learned that your face, neck, décolletage, shoulders, and upper back had to match. Think of a marble bust in a museum. "From the dinner table up" also refers to your arms, elbows, and hands. Skeletal hands with papery skin and bulging blue veins and elephant-skin elbows can be a stark contrast with the fresh and glowing face you have been conscientiously maintaining. You have to walk to that dinner table, so your knees, thighs, and feet are part of the picture. Sagging knees and dry, cracked heels will definitely detract from your overall look. The effect is jarring. The difference might make others wonder just why your face clashes with your body.

No one wants to cover up all the time. Leggings and pants hide crepey knees, three-quarter-length sleeves conceal shar-pei elbows, and sensible shoes camouflage bony feet, but having fewer fashion restrictions will make you look and feel younger and pep up your style. Cellulite should not keep you from being seen in a bathing suit without a wrap or cover-up. No matter how well you take care of your face, a body that shows too much wear and tear ages you.

Age spots, skin tags, cellulite, bumps on the upper arms, dark, rough elbows and knees, and cracked heels are normal parts of aging. Your body inexplicably starts growing things—orange-peel and chicken skin, rough, scaly patches, random bumps and spots, and deep creases. These degradations of time happen to just about everyone. With age, your immune system gets sluggish, and irregularities slip through. You can boost cell metabolism with the Lancer Anti-Aging Method for Body.

Your entire body needs more care as you get older. You have to work harder to maintain yourself, because problems snowball at a faster clip the older you are. The earlier you take care of a new, unwanted development, the more easily you can correct it before it gets worse. The Lancer Anti-Aging Method for Body will improve the texture of your skin and make the tone uniform in just five minutes a day. If you take care of your entire body early enough, maintenance is a breeze. If you are late to the party, you can reverse the changes and slow down further deterioration.

Everyone Needs Body Care

A gorgeous twenty-seven-year-old actress was sent to see me by her agent. She had just had a major break. In three months' time, she was going to have a leading role in a big film to be shot at an exotic location over a six-month period. She was to play a fifteen-year-old. The instructions from her agent: Take care of everything. He did not want to see smile lines, and her entire body had to look pristine.

Her Mediterranean skin was flawless. To make her look younger than her age, total skin care was in order. Every inch of her had to be bright, supple, and fresh. She did the Lancer Anti-Aging Method and the Lancer Anti-Aging Method for Body for the full three months leading up to the film. We focused on her hands, elbows, and knees to make her look newly minted. By the time she was ready to leave for location, she was a vision of vibrant youth—breathtaking.

The Takeaway: It does not take long to see your skin respond to the Lancer Method, but the improvements in your face will be the fastest.

A DIFFERENT LANDSCAPE

The skin on your body is very different from the skin on your face, neck, and chest. In fact, the skin of your face alone has dozens of variations. The thickness of the epidermis, the vascular structure, the cell organization, the sebaceous glands, pores, and a host of other characteristics are remarkably diverse from one inch of the body to the next. For example, simply by studying skin cells found under the nails of a rape victim, forensic scientists can identify what part of the criminal's body the cells came from. They can pinpoint the original location of the cells so well that they are able to say, "Look for a man with scratches on the left side of his neck." There are worlds of difference from your forehead to your heels and a great variation among people. This complexity helps to explain why what works for the skin of some people does not for others.

When shifting from your face, neck, and décolletage to your body, you are dealing with very different skin. The face improves faster than the neck or décolletage. Changes that can be seen in a month on facial skin can take two or three months on the neck and chest. Body skin is tougher than the skin you are treating with the Lancer Method. The skin south of your jawline is less forgiving of injury than your facial skin, mostly because blood circulation is different and skin appendages differ. Since the skin of the body heals more slowly than the face, it will take longer for the Lancer Anti-Aging Method for Body to show results—an average of six months. Different areas have different biological responses at rates that vary. Not all procedures can be performed on all parts of the body, because healing is so unpredictable.

Since the requirements for treating the skin below the bustline are different, you have to use products designed for that purpose if you want to improve the skin all over your body. My full-body regimen uses the principles of the three-step anti-aging method from the last chapter. In order to rejuvenate, you polish, cleanse, and nourish the skin on your body that's likely to show aging. Before introducing you to my full-body regimen, which I explain in detail later in the chapter, I want to review the areas of your body that need your attention as you age.

HOT SPOTS

Certain parts of your body are especially vulnerable to changes that occur over time. Gravity, friction, movement, exposure, and physical stress are all part of the territory. If you neglect these hot spots, you will look timeworn. The Lancer

Anti-Aging Method for Body will simplify taking care of all your aging zones without the need for shelves of special lotions, treatments, and equipment. One method fits all when it comes to improving the texture of your skin from head to toe, because it is based on what the body does naturally to restore itself. The three-step program of polish, cleanse, and nourish with products formulated for use on the body (see page 67) will go a long way toward preventing and correcting annoying signs of aging.

Take care of your body with the Lancer Method every day for six months and see how your skin improves. Take a photo of yourself and close-ups of problem areas when you begin. Reshoot the same areas every month. See how far your skin has come.

Before discussing the program, some hot spot troubleshooting is in order. From the arms and hands to the torso and butt to the legs and feet, every inch of your body deserves to be pampered, softened, and smoothed.

Hands

Your hands show your age. A loss of collagen and elastin leads to less volume, which means veins that bulge become visible. Older hands are skeletonized, with every bone and tendon on display. Age spots that appear as the result of sun damage from years of exposure become evident. Polishing each day will stimulate collagen production and fade age spots.

Do not use harsh soaps or liquid soap containing alcohol on your hands. Use a gentle cleanser with AHA to correct hyperpigmentation. Always nourish your skin after washing your hands. Using sunscreen religiously will prevent the debut of new spots. If your dark spots have not faded enough, consult with a dermatologist about advanced fluorescent pulsed-light technology to remove them.

If your hands are dry, particularly during cold weather, you should try an intensive at-home treatment. Slather your hands with the nourishing cream and an anti-aging stem cell product at night and wear white cotton gloves to bed. The products will penetrate while you sleep, and your hands will be soft and supple when you remove the gloves in the morning.

Elbows

Not the most attractive part of the body, elbows are knobby and awkward. The folds and creases of your elbow skin are there for a purpose. Without that extra skin, you would not be able to bend your arm. When you hold your arms straight, the elbow skin bunches up. Elbows are often the first place dryness and flakiness appear. Elbows lack the sebaceous glands that keep the rest of your skin lubricated, which is why the skin on the joints can look like dry elephant skin. That sandpaper-dry skin can be so rough that it snags long sleeves.

Always use sunscreen on your elbows, because the sun will darken dry skin faster than the rest of your body, making them even more noticeable. If your elbows become very scaly and dry, blister, bleed, crust, or hurt, check with a dermatologist to be certain the problem is not psoriasis or eczema.

Avoid leaning on tables or other hard surfaces with your elbows and forearms. The pressure and friction can worsen their condition, creating a callus that is darker than the surrounding skin. Do not pick off dead skin. Polishing each day will take care of that. Nourishing twice a day will rehydrate the area. If your elbows sting and burn, try using a cool compress to quiet them.

Polishing each day will slough off the dead cells that get trapped in the creases of your elbows and stimulate cell renewal. A good cleanser will continue exfoliating and prepare the dry skin to drink in the moisturizing ingredients in the nourish step. With the Lancer Anti-Aging Method for Body, problem elbows are covered.

Chicken Skin

The red bumps that can crop up in patches on the backs of your arms, your thighs, and your derriere are called keratosis pilaris. These can range from small pinkish-to-red bumps that are not irritated to red, inflamed bumps. Since about 50 percent of those affected have a family history, keratosis pilaris is largely thought to be a genetic disorder. The disorder affects 50 to 80 percent of adolescents and 40 percent of adults.

Those bumpy, red spots are the result of pores clogged with keratin that become inflamed. Exfoliation to unclog pores is an effective treatment, so the polish step should do the job. AHA (alpha hydroxy acid) will do the surface work, and BHA (beta hydroxy acid) salicylic acid goes deeper with anti-microbial properties to fight bacteria and inflammation. Do not scrub your skin when you exfoliate or cleanse, because that will only aggravate the inflammation. If the exfoliation process is not enough, talk to your dermatologist about prescribed ammonium lactate cream or lotions, retinoids, and corticosteroids.

Skin Tags

Moving to the trunk, we see skin tags, affectionately called the barnacles of aging. A skin tag or acrochordon is a small benign tumor that looks like a piece of hanging skin. They appear mostly in areas where skin rubs against skin, like the armpits, under the breasts, and on the groin, chest, neck, and eyelids. They commonly occur in skin creases or folds. Skin tags have a core of fibers and ducts, nerve cells, fat cells, and an epidermis. Susceptibility is partly inherited. People who are overweight, pregnant, and diabetic are more prone to develop skin tags.

Initially, skin tags are small and flattened like a pinhead bump. Exfoliating every day at this stage can make them disappear painlessly. In their infancy, skin tags will respond to topical treatments. If you have skin tags that are unsightly nuisances, see a dermatologist to have them removed. Your dermatologist will know if it's a tag or something more important.

Legs

If you shave your legs, you are exfoliating them. With the Lancer Anti-Aging Method for Body, you will exfoliate two more times, with the body polish and the body cleanse steps of my program; nourishing is then step three. Extremities tend to get dry. Your legs will enjoy all the benefits of the Lancer Method's controlled injury. If you have not protected your legs with sunscreen or have had bad sunburns, you might have sun damage in the form of age spots. The Lancer Method is formulated to help fade those dark spots and improve the texture of the skin on your legs.

Knees

The fashion for bare legs has revealed that some of the great beauties of our time have saggy, unattractive knees. Knees sag, get crepey, and develop "kninkles," deep creases and wrinkles, not to mention frontal cellulite. Knee sag can affect anyone, regardless of weight. The laxity in the skin also stems from the natural loss of collagen, elastin, and muscle mass that occurs with age. Like the elbows, your knees work hard. The skin of your knees is forced to bend and stretch constantly, which can cause laxity. In certain positions, your knees have to support the weight of your entire body. Knees are rarely the focus of anti-aging treatments, but there are steps you can take to prevent their aging in an unsightly way and to transform an often less-than-perfect body part.

The low concentration of sebaceous glands in that area is responsible for the dryness that ages knees prematurely. Knee skin therapy can make big improvements. Exfoliating your knees every day will revitalize them on a cellular level. Nourishing your skin to moisturize and to stimulate collagen production helps, too. Exercise can build muscles that lift the sag and fill out crepey areas in the fleshy part of the knee. Yoga and Pilates will keep your knees strong and flexible.

Surgical knee lifts should be avoided. They are expensive and leave a large scar that can spread because of the knee's movement. The scars can become thick, raised, and darker than the surrounding skin. Skin tightening procedures are a better option if your problem is severe.

Cellulite

Orange-peel syndrome. Cottage cheese skin. Hail damage. These are just a few of the wonderful, descriptive labels for cellulite, the dreaded dimpled, lumpy appearance seen on the backs of the thighs, along with the butt, knees, stomach, and upper arms of close to 90 percent of women and many men. You do not have to be overweight to have cellulite. You cannot imagine how much airbrushing is done to photographs of famous limbs. Cellulite becomes more prevalent with age, as the skin loses elasticity.

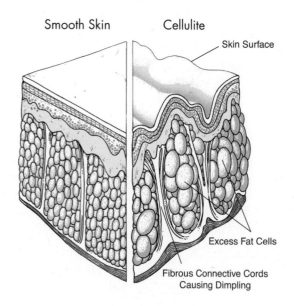

Cellulite is the result of unevenness of fatty tissue beneath the skin's surface. The bumpy appearance is created when fat pushes against connective cords called septa that attach the skin to the underlying muscle. As fat cells accumulate, they push up against the skin's surface, while the connective tissue pulls down, causing the skin above to pucker.

There is no clear-cut cause for cellulite, but there are many theories.

- Genetics do play a role. Certain genes have been identified that may predispose a person to developing dimpled skin. Some of the inherited characteristics include slow metabolism, the way fat is distributed under the skin, and insufficient circulation.

- Hormonal factors are involved, particularly estrogen and the hormones associated with stress.
- Lifestyle issues are a key contributor. A diet full of fat, simple carbohydrates, salt, and too little fiber is likely to lead to greater amounts of cellulite.
- Chronic dehydration and yo-yo dieting influence how much cellulite you have.
- Cellulite may be more pronounced in smokers, inactive people, and those who stand or sit in one position for long periods.
- Cellulite tends to be less visible on darker skin.

Reduce the Appearance of Cellulite

The Lancer Anti-Aging Method for Body works to improve the appearance of cellulite by making your skin more taut and elastic, which reduces the appearance of dimpling. Beware the claims of cellulite creams, which have not been proven effective. Caffeine in topical form is an ingredient that seems to have a slight beneficial effect.

There are a number of therapeutic treatments used to improve cellulite: lymphatic massage and heat therapy, ultrasound, radio frequency therapy, radial wave therapy, electrical stimulation that tightens the skin, and surgery. I have used fillers in some stubborn cases. Before trying any of these treatments, you should use the Lancer Method to take your skin as far as it can go. Even the most stubborn cases improve in time. If you persist, you will see a difference.

Feet

Your feet take a beating. Not only do they carry you all day, but for the women out there, your feet are often squeezed into high-heeled, pointy shoes worn without stockings. Shoes that are too loose are equally damaging. The friction in the areas that do not bear weight causes corns and blisters. Calluses form on the weight-bearing soles of the feet and heels. The best defense for keeping your feet in good shape is not to wear the same shoes every day. Vary the height of the heel and the style of the shoe.

Polishing your feet when you shower or bathe will help to keep your feet soft and even-toned. I do not recommend using pumice stones, because it's difficult to clean them well enough to stop the growth of bacteria. Buffing your feet every day and taking care of them with a pedicure every other week should be enough to soften your feet and erase signs of wear and tear. Here are some tips to keep your feet healthy:

- Apply sunscreen to the tops of your feet and to your ankles every day.
- Be sure to polish heels, soles, and toes daily.
- Whenever your feet are wet, dry them thoroughly—especially between the toes—to avoid athlete's foot. Wipe moisturizer or cream from between your toes as well.
- Wear flip-flops in locker rooms or when walking on damp floors.
- Rotate your shoes to prevent repeated pinching and rubbing in the same places.
- Use cushioning insoles in your shoes.
- To give your feet an intense moisturizing treatment, lavishly apply stem cell moisturizer on your feet and wear white cotton socks to bed. Absorbing the anti-aging treatment, your feet will heal as you sleep.

When you wear sandals, you want your feet to look elegant, not battered. If you work on it, you can improve the appearance of your feet. If you have neglected them and your feet are a mess, make an appointment with a podiatrist to see what can be done to correct any problems you might have.

Nails Are Skin, Too

Nails are made of hardened keratin, the same protein found in skin and hair, and are produced by cells in the fingers and toes. Your fingernails grow on average twice as fast as your toenails. Just as the appearance of your skin is a window into your health, your nails reflect what is going on inside you. This is why nail problems increase with age. Though nearly everyone has injured a nail, had an ingrown toenail, or experienced a fungal infection at one time or another, changes in the color, shape, or thickness of your nails, as well as swelling, bleeding, or pain, can signal serious health problems, including heart, liver, thyroid, or kidney disease, diabetes, or anemia.

A dermatologist is trained to identify the symptoms revealed by your nails. As broad examples, splinter hemorrhages—thin reddish brown lines under the nails—may be a sign of heart disease. If you see a dark discoloration that involves the cuticle, melanoma, a malignant form of skin cancer, could be an issue. If you notice changes in your nails—texture, color, rippling, bumps, pits, curling—check with your dermatologist. Nail changes can indicate a serious medical condition that you will want to know about.

To keep your nails healthy, apply moisturizer to them every day, especially the cuticles. Do not pick at your cuticles and hangnails. Do not cut cuticles. Soften them with nourisher and push them back. Break the habit of biting or chewing on your nails. Reducing stress and anxiety would make breaking this habit easier. You should give yourself or have a high-quality manicure/pedicure every other week. If you have professional manicures and pedicures, invest in your own nail care equipment rather than risk an infection. Only a podiatrist or chiropodist should use a blade on your feet. A foot file after a soak should be adequate to soften calluses and corns. Always be certain your toenails are cut short and straight across, because curved nails can become ingrown. If you develop an ingrown nail, do not try to fix it. See a dermatologist to avoid a bad infection.

Old Hair Day

Those gray hairs that start popping up during the thirties are one of the first signs of aging. As you age, your hair follicles produce less melanin, and your hair color becomes lighter. Your body is producing less keratin, the protein that makes hair healthy and strong. Without enough keratin, hair strands become thinner, more porous, and brittle. As a consequence, hair becomes finer and thinner for most people from the age of thirty on. Part of the reason for this change is that the growth rate of hair slows down, and hair that has been shed is replaced more slowly. This process affects your eyelashes as well. Not only do they break as they get increasingly brittle, but they replenish more slowly.

Hormone fluctuations during menopause can contribute to hair loss. Since estrogen levels are diminished, androgens or male hormones can thin hair where you want it and cause facial hair to grow where you do not. For men with a genetic susceptibility to baldness, testosterone is converted to DHT, a more potent form of the male hormone, which binds to cells in hair follicles and eventually kills them.

Aside from a loss of density, the texture of hair changes with age. Hair becomes drier and coarser as sebum production slows down by an estimated 10 percent every decade. Sebum lubricates the hair as well as the skin. The combination of chronological age, damaging environmental exposure, professional-grade hot styling tools, and dyeing and straightening chemicals can decimate your hair. Dull, brittle, frayed, and parched strands result.

Lifestyle plays a big role in the health of your hair. Stress can make your tresses lifeless, just as it does your skin. Whether you have been working overtime to finish a project or are taking care of your aging parents and teenage kids, your stress revs up the production of hormones that lead to inflammation. The inflammation can compromise your scalp's barrier function. Hair care products you have been using can suddenly cause stinging, tingling, and itching sensations because your hair and scalp have become drier and the chemicals in the products are penetrating deeper into your skin, creating a reaction.

Mother Nature Is Rarely Wrong

Chris McMillan of Chris McMillan Salon is a renowned Beverly Hills stylist. He created Jennifer Aniston's iconic *Friends* hairstyle and has worked with her ever since. He has transformed the standards of red-carpet hair with his loose, low-key aesthetic. You have seen his work on the covers of all the major magazines—*Vogue*, *Harper's Bazaar*, *Vanity Fair*, *InStyle*, *Rolling Stone*, *GQ*. His philosophy on hair color is in sync with my message about taking it slow and keeping it natural:

> I am a believer that the hair color you are born with tends to be the most complementary to your skin tone. I personally don't think that Mother Nature got it wrong for all of us! For instance, look at pictures from your childhood when your hair was in its most natural state and before it had been altered. You don't look at those pictures and think to yourself, *If only I had darkened my base a little I would have been a more attractive kid.* Quite the contrary. How often do we look back and wish we could go back to our natural, healthy, unprocessed hair?
>
> When consulting with my clients, I always recommend that they refer back to when they were babies. Notice that when we, as adults, start to color our hair, typically we start with highlights. A highlight is really just an enhancement of one's own natural base color. We don't chemically alter the entire body of hair. As we progress, and we start to see that change is possible, that's when we start to consider more dramatic color overhauls. Only two types of people alter their overall color: those looking to cover gray, and those looking to produce a dramatic effect. Those looking to cover gray should always stick to a color as close to their natural as possible, which again lends to the notion that what we are born with is generally our most complementary, "natural" look, then simultaneously begin to make other changes to compensate for the new hair color (think changing makeup colors or tanning), thereby making for a more authentic look. Beauty should look effortless and classic! Use Mother Nature as your guide. She's rarely wrong.

Every strand of hair is its own universe with its own sweat gland, a sebaceous gland, muscle, and circulatory system. With stress, each follicle becomes tight and rigid, because stress spikes the production of adrenaline, which converts to androgens that make hair fall out. Chronic stress leads to irregularities in insulin production, which ends up inflaming your entire body. Severe psychological or physical stress, such as divorce, surgery, or the death of a loved one, can cause hair loss, either by making hair fall out as with alopecia areata, or with telogen effluvium, a condition that pushes growing hairs into a resting phase. Extreme weight loss can reduce hormone production, which can lead to hair thinning as well. See a dermatologist if you notice unusual hair loss when combing or washing your hair, because sudden, excessive hair loss can signal an underlying medical condition.

Certain medications and supplements can lead to extensive hair loss. Anticoagulants such as warfarin, anti-depressants, oral contraceptives, and medications for arthritis and blood pressure are among the commonly prescribed medicines that can thin your hair.

One way to keep your hair strong and shiny is to consume nutrients that will promote hair health. What you eat helps to fortify the hair follicles and the scalp that surrounds them. Protein consumption is essential for healthy hair. People who do not get enough protein in their diets will slow the rate of new hair growth. As hair is naturally shed, it will not grow back as quickly.

I have taken you on a comprehensive tour of the aging zones of your body. Now I will teach you how to have beautiful skin from head to toe.

THE LANCER ANTI-AGING METHOD
FOR BODY

A few years ago, I believe that Jay Leno referred to me on air as "the doctor who polishes the breasts of Hollywood." That statement is true—only figuratively, of course. The Lancer Anti-Aging Method for Body takes advantage of the same process of self-repair as the Lancer Method. You will be doing the three steps— polish, cleanse, and nourish—each day from head to toe. When you do the Lancer Anti-Aging Method for Body, you will exfoliate your entire body whenever you bathe or shower to stimulate your skin to act young by tapping into its innate healing power. You will boost cell renewal and promote collagen and elastin production when you buff your body, just as you do when you polish your face, neck, and décolletage. Then you will cleanse, which will exfoliate as well as wash away dead cells, dirt, and excess oil. You will nourish your skin with a treatment cream that will not only moisturize and smooth but also fight the destructive action of free radicals and deliver needed oxygen to skin cells.

To put the brakes on signs of aging all over your body, polishing is essential. Unless you live in a tropical paradise, a good portion of your skin is usually not exposed to the elements. The good news is that your unexposed skin should be in reasonably good shape. Using this three-step program will keep it that way. For your hands, arms, legs, and feet that see the light of day, exfoliating will help to correct sun damage, even skin tone, and postpone some signs of skin aging. You will follow by cleansing and nourishing to texturize and tone your skin.

The Lancer Anti-Aging Method for Body

Polish your body whenever you shower or bathe. I do not recommend using loofahs, body puffs, or shower gloves unless they are laundered with each use. Wet mechanical exfoliators are a breeding ground for bacteria. The exfoliants in your polish will do the job.

Follow with the body cleanse.
    Use body nourish after you bathe and/or before you go to bed.
    Apply sunscreen to hands, forearms, legs, feet, and any other exposed areas in the morning.

Body Polish

Your first step is to polish your skin. Your goal is to remove dry, dead skin cells, excess oils, and residue to reveal smoother, younger-looking skin. Polishing your body from head to toe will revitalize your skin and make it soft to the touch.

- Apply a moderate amount of exfoliant to dry skin with dry hands.
- Segment your body: Start with one foot and work up to your knee, then repeat on the other leg, massaging in a gentle circular motion with wet hands. Spend a minute a leg.
- Work your hand, forearm, upper arm, and shoulder on each arm for a minute.
- Pay special attention to your aging zones—hands, elbows, back of your thighs, knees, heels, toes and between them. Anywhere you see roughness, scaling, sun damage, or sags, dimples, and wrinkles needs to be buffed.
- Rinse with lukewarm water and pat dry. Make sure you wash away all the fine grains of the body buff.

Recommended Body Scrubs

You should look for a body buff that contains mechanical and chemical exfoliants as well as anti-oxidants and anti-inflammatory agents.

Luxury:

Lancer Skincare The Method: Body Polish

La Prairie Cellular Mineral Body Exfoliator

Sisley-Paris Energizing Foaming Exfoliant

Moderate:

Kiehl's Lavender Gently Exfoliating Body Scrub

Clinique Sparkle Skin Body Exfoliator

Affordable:

Dove Gentle Exfoliating Body Wash with NutriumMoisture

Burt's Bees Radiance Exfoliating Body Wash

Body Cleanse

Wash your body in the same order you buff your skin and rinse well. Avoid washcloths and bathing mitts, because bacteria will grow in them if you do not launder with each use.

Recommended Body Cleansers

Select a cleanser with a chemical exfoliant. The cleanser should be soothing for dry skin.

Luxury:

Lancer Skincare The Method: Body Cleanse

Erno Laszlo Sea Mud Deep Cleansing Bar

La Prairie Cellular Energizing Bath and Shower Gelee

Moderate:

Kiehl's Coriander Bath & Shower Liquid Body Cleanser

Clinique Deep Comfort Body Wash

Affordable:

Dove VisibleCare Radiance Crème Body Wash

Aveeno Stress Relief Body Wash

Body Nourish

Moisturizing your entire body after you bathe will delay signs of aging and improve texture and tone. Applying nourisher while your skin is damp will make absorption of active ingredients more effective.

- Apply liberally to aging zones—elbows, heels, knees.
- Be sure to dry between your toes and do not moisturize.

Recommended Body Moisturizers

A good moisturizer should contain anti-oxidants, skin tighteners, AHAs, and oxygenating liposomes.

Luxury:

Lancer Skincare The Method: Body Nourish

Chanel Crème Lissante Jeunesse et Fermeté (Firming and Rejuvenating Cream)

AmorePacific Moisture Bound Vitalizing Body Lotion

Moderate:

Kiehl's Deluxe Hand & Body Lotion with Aloe Vera & Oatmeal

Clinique Deep Comfort Body Butter

Affordable:

Eucerin Skin Calming Daily Moisturizing Creme

Aveeno Daily Moisturizing Lotion

LOOK FOR THE "UGLY DUCKLINGS" IN YOUR SELF-EXAM

Skin cancer is the most common form of cancer in the United States. There are more new cases of skin cancer each year than the combined numbers of breast, prostate, lung, and colon cancer cases. Since one in five Americans will develop skin cancer in his or her lifetime, you need to be aware of the signs and symptoms so that you can have a dermatologist check any moles or marks you suspect.

Though skin cancer comes in many forms, there are three main types you should know about.

Basal Cell Skin Cancer

This is the most common skin cancer in people with light complexions. It starts in the basal cells of the epidermis. It is rare in people with dark skin. This is what to look for:

- A small, smooth bump that is fleshy and might have an indentation in the middle
- A bump that bleeds, crusts over, and repeats the cycle

- A tender, flat, red spot that bleeds easily
- A firm scar-like lesion

Squamous Cell Skin Cancer

These tumors appear most often on sun-exposed areas. The forehead, nose, ears, lower lip, hands, and hairline are places where squamous cell skin cancer is commonly found. This type of cancer can occur on areas of the skin that have been burned or exposed to chemicals or radiation therapy. Squamous cell carcinoma can grow large rapidly and can spread to nearby lymph nodes. Though rare for dark-skinned people, this form of cancer is number two for light skin tones. Here are the first signs:

- A firm red bump
- A scaly patch of skin or growth that bleeds or develops a crust
- A sore that fails to heal

Melanoma

This is a serious, malignant form of skin cancer that can spread to bones and organs. Melanoma begins in the melanocytes in the basal level of the epidermis. As you will remember, melanocytes produce the pigment melanin, which protects deeper layers of the skin from sun damage. Melanoma runs in families. The cancer develops when harmful UV rays from the sun damage skin cells. A change in the size, shape, or color of a mole or other skin growth is the first sign to look for. Be on the alert for these changes:

- A thickening or rising of a mole that had been flat
- Scaling, bleeding, oozing, erosion, or crusting of the surface
- Swelling, redness, or small new patches of color around the surrounding skin
- Burning, tickling, or itching
- Softening or small pieces breaking off

Women have been educated about the importance of self-examination for early detection in breast cancer. Everyone—both men and women—has to become equally aware of the early signs and symptoms of skin cancer. You should give yourself an exam once a month to look for any changes or new lesions.

The "Ugly Duckling" concept will help you to identify possible melanomas. The idea is that melanomas look different compared with surrounding moles or freckles. Unaffected moles look like each other, but a cancerous lesion looks and feels different from other marks on your skin. The ABCDE rule has been developed to evaluate skin changes and identify melanomas:

A—Asymmetry: If you draw a line through the mole, the two halves will not match.

B—Border: The borders of an early melanoma are often uneven. The edges may have notches or scallops.

C—Color: When a mole or mark develops a variety of colors—shades of brown, tan, or black—consider the change a warning sign. Red, blue, or another color might appear.

D—Diameter: Melanomas are usually larger across than the eraser on the end of a pencil, about a quarter inch, but can be smaller when first noticed.

E—Evolution: Any change in size, shape, color, or elevation—or any new symptom such as bleeding, crusting, or itching—requires examination by a dermatologist.

If your dermatologist finds skin cancer, the growth will be biopsied to determine what sort of cancer it is and how it should be handled.

Skin Cancer Is Easy to Miss

A Hollywood leading man, who is a patient, gave his publicist a gift certificate for services at my office. She was fair-skinned, in her mid-fifties, and what I would call a head-to-toe derma-dilemma. She had not taken very good care of her skin. When I handed her the mirror and Q-tip, she was concerned about her neck and her softening jawline.

While giving her a total body skin exam, I found three cancerous skin tumors. One was on her back, one inside her knee, and another on the side of her left breast. She and other doctors who had examined her had assumed the lesions were sun spots. A dermatologist would not have missed that cancer. This is an important reason to see a dermatologist regularly, at least once a year. If caught early enough, skin cancer can be managed without too much fuss.

The Takeaway: Examine the skin on your entire body carefully once a month for cancer signs. Do not forget your back. Maybe a loved one can help if you are having difficulty.

*   *   *

You are set with a plan for your face, neck, and chest and another for your entire body. You will see progress if you use the Lancer Method every day. If you fall off the wagon, hop right back on. Do not let your skin go back to sleep. If you are like most of my patients, the improvements you see in your skin will motivate you to stick to the program. You will know it's worth it when people notice a difference. They will ask you what you have changed or if you have been on vacation, because you have the Lancer Glow.

In the following chapters, you will learn how to tweak the Lancer Method for supercharged anti-aging, acne treatment, rosacea relief, and sensitive skin—the four basic groups of skin care. These conditions all fall on a continuum of inflammation. To understand the specific courses of treatment within the Lancer Method, it is helpful to know more about the Lancer Ethnicity Scale. Many of your skin concerns are inherited from your ancestors, and your heritage determines the way in which your skin responds to treatments.

Part Two

FINE-TUNING THE LANCER ANTI-AGING METHOD

5

Looking at Your Family Tree

When I meet new patients, my recommendations for their treatment are based on much more than just their appearance. I always ask my patients about their ancestry as far back as they know, and specifically where their maternal and paternal grandparents are from. In our global society, borders are melting. We live in a world of mixed ancestry. A green-eyed redhead with pale, freckled skin might have an ancestor from Portugal, Spain, or Morocco with a dark complexion. An African American might have a Swedish grandmother with pale skin and hair. The amount of pigmentation in the skin is not necessarily an accurate reflection of genetic ancestry. Fair skin can behave like dark skin, and dark skin can react like light skin depending on your genetic makeup. The complexity of skin types is far more than meets the eye. Look around at your family reunion, study an old family album, and talk to your relatives. Your blood relatives may exhibit a broad spectrum of skin tones. You may have forgotten or never known that your British great-grandmother married an East Indian, but you could be carrying genes for darker skin.

I had my revelation about the importance of understanding a patient's ethnic origins back in 1997. I was attending a national conference in Boston, where one panel featured prominent, highly respected dermatologists talking about poor outcomes from resurfacing techniques. I listened to my colleagues review complications from simple laser procedures. They reported that some patients had inexplicably developed second- and third-degree burns from laser or chemical treatments that had left other patients with exemplary results. An unlucky few were in the burn unit for months, requiring hyperbaric oxygen to heal their burns and reconstructive work to repair their skin.

Just as pigmentation or the color of skin is inherited, the way wounds heal, even the controlled injury of laser treatment, is determined by genetics. We know that what works for Northern European blue-eyed blondes might not necessarily be an effective treatment for darker-complected people of African, Middle Eastern, Mediterranean, Asian, East Indian, or American Indian descent. Thinking about my clinical observations, it occurred to me that without knowing patients' ancestry, we could subject them to treatments with unpredictable outcomes that might damage their skin.

On the flight home, I had finished my reading and pulled the in-air magazine from the seat pocket to flip through. I stopped at the map of the world showing the routes the airline flew, which I studied. As I did, I thought about dividing up the world in terms of geographic global ancestry. The name of the country is not important, but the global geographic location is. The map of geographic skin pigmentation I envisioned is on the next page.

There seem to be as many skin tones as there are people—the variation is that broad. Skin color and hair color are created by the amount, type, and packaging of the pigment melanin, all of which are determined genetically. We know little about the genetic basis of pigmentation. Rather than a specific skin color gene, many genes work together to produce your skin tone. Ethnic skin coloration has a lot to do with geography and evolution. Skin variations in ethnicity differ not only in color but also in skin components, including collagen, elastin, blood vessels, lymphatics, nerve fiber, glandular components, immunity, and reactivity. No precise standard exists! Treatment approach requires caution... always.

HUMAN SKIN COLOR DISTRIBUTION

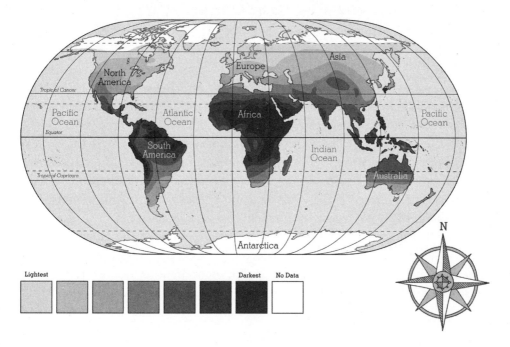

LIFE UNDER THE SUN

Different skin tones developed as adaptations to geography and the sun's ultraviolet rays. As you already know, melanin has an important physiological role in protecting the skin from sun damage. The closer our ancient ancestors were to the equator, the more melanin was needed to protect their skin.

Ultraviolet rays help the body use vitamin D to absorb the calcium needed for strong bones, but too much exposure to ultraviolet rays can strip away folate, a nutrient essential for fetal development. Skin pigment developed as the body's way of balancing the need for vitamin D and the need for folate. Darker skin evolved close to the equator to prevent folate deficiency. The cardinal rule is that evolution favors reproductive success. When groups migrated farther from the equator where ultraviolet rays are lower, natural selection favored lighter skin to allow enough vitamin-D-forming UV rays to penetrate. Today pigmentation varies within geographic regions, but there is still a strong correlation between the strength of the sun's UV rays and skin pigmentation.

WHY DARKER SKIN LOOKS YOUNGER LONGER THAN FAIR SKIN AND OTHER ETHNIC DIFFERENCES

Your pigmentation depends on the quantity and quality of melanin in your skin, the amount of UV exposure you have, and genetics. Melanin is the natural skin pigment that protects skin cells from UV rays. Melanocytes produce melanin, which is packaged in melanosomes—found mostly in the basal level—to protect the germinating epidermal cells from UV damage. Though concentrated in the basal layer, melanosomes are dispersed throughout the epidermis. More melanosomes are concentrated in the epidermis of the head and forearms than the rest of the body. Everyone has approximately the same number of epidermal melanosomes, but their size and distribution differ with ethnicity and different shades of skin. The melanosomes in darkly pigmented skin are larger and more individually dispersed compared with other skin tones. In fairer-skinned people, the melanosomes are smaller and are grouped in complexes of two or more. The most

---

The Princess and the Pea

A stunning young Eurasian woman was waiting for me in a treatment room. At first glance, her skin was close to flawless. No sun damage was observable. Her complexion was pale, slightly sallow, and even-toned; and her pores were imperceptible. This patient obviously took great care to maintain her skin.

When I asked her what I could do for her, she pointed to a fine dark brown line about three inches long on her jawline that could easily be overlooked because of its position. She had lightly scratched her face with a fingernail months earlier. Instead of healing, the faint, superficial red line turned dark brown.

I was not surprised when she told me her ancestors were Swiss, African American, and Chinese. Her genetics explained the hyperpigmentation response to the injury. Skin with high levels of melanin reacts to the inflammation caused by injury by producing more pigment in an effort to protect the skin. This response may cause dark spots and blotchiness. This woman was definitely not a candidate for laser treatments in the future. Medical restoration was the only answer.

The Takeaway: Looks can be deceptive. Skin genetics are complex, and you never know what traits are present in your genes. Without considering your ancestry, you will not be able to identify potential problems before they develop.

lightly pigmented types have about half as much melanin as skin that is darkly pigmented, leaving fair skin more vulnerable to the damaging effects of sunlight.

Since melanin is built-in SPF (sun protection factor), skin pigmentation dictates skin changes associated with photo-aging. More darkly pigmented skin begins to show signs of aging later than lightly pigmented skin. Though fair complexions tend to wrinkle and sag earlier, darkly pigmented skin can become mottled, hyperpigmented, hypopigmented, or generally uneven in tone when injured or inflamed.

Some researchers have found that on average the darkest skin tones contain more corneocyte layers in the stratum corneum than the fairest skin, though there is no difference in the thickness of the layers. The cell layers are more compact in the darkest skin, which creates greater cohesion among the cells. This compressed architecture of the stratum corneum strengthens the barrier function in darker skin. Very dark skin tends to have larger pores and greater sebum secretion.

THE LANCER ETHNICITY SCALE

Thomas Fitzpatrick, one of my professors at Harvard, developed what is now known as the Fitzpatrick Classification Skin Typing System, which has become the standard method for defining skin pigmentation. He was measuring the skin's ability to tolerate light or UV rays to find the correct dose of UVA for the treatment of psoriasis. He had six skin types: very fair, fair, light golden, olive, brown, and dark brown.

I wanted to build on his concepts of phototype by including heritage as part of the definition. The Lancer Ethnicity Scale, based on geography and heredity, is summarized in the following chart:

The Lancer Ethnicity Scale (LES)

ETHNIC BACKGROUND	LES TYPE
African Background	
Central, East, West African	V
Eritrean and Ethiopian	V
North African, Middle East Arabic	V
Sephardic Jews	IV

ETHNIC BACKGROUND	LES TYPE
Asian Background	
Chinese, Korean, Japanese, Thai, Vietnamese	IV
Filipino, Polynesian	IV
European Background	
European Jews	III
Celtic	I
Central, Eastern European	II
Nordic	I
Northern European	I–II
Southern European, Mediterranean	III–IV
Central/South American Background	
Central/South American Indian	IV
North American Background	
Native American (includes Inuit)	III

There is a simple formula for finding your LES skin type. Just add up the numbers that correspond to your grandparents' ethnicities and divide by four. The higher your score is, the more likely you will experience complications with healing after a cosmetic procedure. A high number indicates you might have an adverse reaction to aggressive resurfacing procedures, including laser treatments

LES SKIN TYPE	RISK
LES I	Very low
LES II	Low
LES III	Moderate
LES IV	Significant
LES V	Considerable

and chemical peels. If there is healing involved, there is risk. Once you calculate your LES skin type, the chart that follows lists the level of risk of an adverse reaction to a resurfacing procedure.

Though I developed the Lancer Ethnicity Scale to predict complications from procedures, the scale can be applied to skin care as well. The LES types provide a green-, yellow-, or red-light approach to treating the skin, whether with topicals or procedures. Depending on your type, your skin will react differently to skin care products. Let me explain.

LES I or II: These types do not get a free pass. Though hyperpigmentation is not a huge problem, fair skin requires gentle care. Not only is fair skin susceptible to sun damage, but it can be highly sensitive and reactive. Dryness and rosacea can be problems. Blood vessels can become hyperactive, resulting in instability. This tendency to be reactive is why I am including a chapter on caring for sensitive skin to avoid premature aging. Of course, sensitivity occurs in all skin types. When skin is hyper-reactive, you have to introduce new products gradually. People with this level of skin pigmentation begin to polish and use anti-aging products gradually to avoid irritating their skin.

LES II or III: These types are deceptive. Skin with this level of pigmentation does not burn quickly, but does develop wrinkles and sagging. LES IIs and IIIs can scar easily, and discoloration can take years to improve. When lightening chemicals quiet a hyperpigmentation reaction, the pigment cells can go dead with this type. The rebound is to less pigmentation or hypopigmentation, which produces white zones. Skin with this level of pigmentation might have to be eased into polishing, because the transportation of signals from the stratum corneum can be aggressive and result in hyperpigmentation.

LES III or IV: Olive-colored skin has to be treated with extreme caution. This skin tone might age slowly, but can easily become inflamed. Olive skin has relatively small pores. The combination of small pores and hyperactive oil glands can lead to acne. Type III or IV skin can discolor with blemishing. People of these skin types can develop dark circles around their eyes. Sometimes skin pigmented at this level only partially responds to color correction. Chapter 7 will present a program for acne-prone or blemished skin.

Do Not Rush into Treatment

A prominent plastic surgeon referred to me a patient who was visiting Beverly Hills from his home in Dubai. One look at his face told me a lot. He obviously had been spending time on his yacht. The pores of his dark skin were enlarged. He was ashen gray and splotchy with dark circles around his eyes. Our conversation about his ancestry revealed that he was a combination of LES III, IV, and V.

He told me he had heard I was the Michelangelo of laser treatments. He was going to be in Beverly Hills for thirty-six hours, and he wanted to get going immediately.

I told him it was not happening. An attempt at a quick fix would only make his skin look worse and could lead to complications that would take months to correct.

This was a man who was used to getting what he wanted. I stood my ground against his protests. I explained that I was just as well known as the skin care guru and assured him that he could improve his skin on an at-home basis without risking injury that could be irreversible. I gave him a protocol that included using products with glycolic acid, vitamin C, stem cells, and retinoids to improve his skin before trying more aggressive procedures. He had to learn the nature of topical skin care to allow his skin to restore itself. His attending staff members took instruction well.

The Takeaway: Olive skin can react in unpredictable ways and should be treated with caution. A quick fix can lead to a slow recovery and permanent damage.

LES V: Black skin, like all other skin types, has great variability. It can be extremely sensitive. If you are not trained to observe the signs, you can miss a reaction. LES V skin can be so sensitive that it becomes severely inflamed in response to even minor irritations. The pigment can become uneven, resulting in hyperpigmentation (increased color) or hypopigmentation (decreased color). Capillaries can become visible, and eyelid folds can become rough. Other common texture changes include scarring—particularly keloids, or raised scars—and depressions in the surface of the skin called pits or divots. Certain ingredients in acne medications or anti-aging products can leave a white or gray film on darkly pigmented skin or lead to inflammation. Special care has to be taken with topicals. The chapters that follow on acne, sensitive skin, and advanced anti-aging will include information of particular interest for people of color.

*　　*　　*

The following chapter takes the basic Lancer Anti-Aging Method to another level of healing and renewal. For some of you, the basic three-step program will be all you need to refresh your skin. If you have been doing the basic Lancer Anti-Aging Method for three to six months and want to do more to stimulate your skin's repair mechanism, you might be ready for the Lancer Advanced Anti-Aging Method. Remember, Lancer Rule Number 1 is not to rush anything. Change takes time.

6

The Lancer Advanced Anti-Aging Method

Now that you have become accustomed to the three steps of the basic Lancer Anti-Aging Method—polish, cleanse, nourish—and are pleased by the improvements you have seen, you might want to boost your skin's healing even further by adding intensive anti-aging steps to your daily regimen. If your skin has suffered sun damage, doing more for your complexion at home will have great benefits. Everyone should do the three-step program for at least a month before taking the treatment up a notch. You have to give your skin time to come to life without overwhelming it. After a month of faithful skin care, you will begin to see your skin brighten. It will be more refined, the texture smoother, and the tone more even. The changes might be dramatic or subtle, but they will be there, leaving you wanting more.

Skin improvements can be compared to losing weight. The more weight you have to lose, the easier it is to take off the pounds, especially at the beginning. If you have not paid much attention to skin care, the improvements that result from my three-step method will be early and striking. If you have done everything in an attempt to stay young, it's as if you have been yo-yo dieting, and you have to work harder to see results. You try the latest product and every procedure you hear about from your friends, but nothing lasts. You struggle to maintain the appearance you have achieved, but it's a slippery slope. If you do not repeat expensive procedures, you end up looking worse than you did before. And I am not even mentioning potential complications from these procedures. At a time when everyone wants a quick fix, it can be difficult to be patient, have faith, and put in the work. You might think, *Why bother with a skin care regimen if a single procedure can correct the problem instantly?* I am here to tell you that any procedure involves a risk. In my years of experience, I have learned that some things work for some people some of the time, and outcomes are not necessarily predictable. That is why I am conservative with my treatment plans.

You Need a Plan to Fight Aging

One morning at ten forty-five a petite forty-six-year-old woman of mixed European ancestry, an LES III to IV, was waiting for me in a treatment room. Her skin looked dusty, and she had first- or second-degree burns on her face. She had made an appointment with a prominent dermatologist for a peel. Though she did not have a regular skin care regimen, her skin was in relatively good shape. Instead of simple skin care, she wanted a quick fix to look her best for her son's wedding.

Her dermatologist gave her a mild, safe, exfoliating peel. First, her skin was cleansed with a glycolic cleanser to remove the oils and corneocytes on the skin's surface. Then the solution was applied. It burns slightly before the acid is neutralized and the solution removed with cold water. The deeper exfoliation normally produces peeling and flaking for three or four days. Within a week, the skin should look healthier and smoother. She was in my office because this did not happen in her case.

After examining the uneven quality of the burns, I realized that the cleaning of her skin before the application of the solution had been inadequate. The saturation of the peel was uneven as a result. The separation of the exfoliated skin cells had been incomplete, leaving textural changes.

She looked as if she had fallen asleep in the sun. Her LES III to IV skin was pitted, crusty, and inflamed. She had daily treatments at the office of her original doctor for a week to moisten, hydrate, and peel away the burned surface. Before seeing me, she had consulted with three other doctors and two aestheticians. The result before my eyes was total "rummage sale" skin.

I had one of my aestheticians use an LED red light treatment to calm the inflammation and instruct her on the three-step program.

I cannot tell you how many times I have seen preventive anti-aging attempts damage the skin of people trying to take care of themselves. Random procedures without a program or plan can result in pitted marks, brown spots, papular inflammatory acne, and skin as thin as cigarette paper. Procedures performed independent of a program are always

risky. You might find yourself struggling to repair your skin and just bring it back to neutral. You need a plan and an approach to fight aging. Do not enter the anti-aging arena by trying a procedure right away. The Lancer Method will prepare your skin to maximize the benefits of any treatments you choose in the future. This is true for the entire skin surface, not just the face.

The Takeaway: A dermatologist can put together a personalized menu for you that will combine products and treatments to take your skin step-by-step to the best it can be. Don't push the process too fast.

ADDING MORE TREATMENT TO YOUR DAILY REGIMEN

Sensitive Skin Warning

If you have acne, rosacea, or sensitive skin, read this chapter for general anti-aging information. Do not introduce new products until you have read the chapter for your condition. Your programs and basic products will be different from the Lancer Advanced Anti-Aging Method.

You are about to expand your at-home treatment beyond the use of sunblock.

The type of skin care products you will gradually add to your daily routine are:

- Keratolytics that enhance the penetration of the other products you are using and make your skin feel smoother.
- Anti-oxidants to minimize the breakdown of collagen and protect the DNA of the keratinocytes.

- Retinoids to increase the production of collagen and elastin, restore cell renewal timing, and even out pigmentation.
- Lightening agents to neutralize and even out your skin color.
- Peptides, a very expensive skin care ingredient, contribute to the skin's structural strength.
- Surrounded by confusion and controversy, stem cells are the new frontier in skin care. Stem cells are undifferentiated or "blank" cells that have the potential to develop into a variety of cell types that carry out different functions. Most cells in the human body are built to function in a particular organ system and to carry out a specific function. Stem cells can replenish their numbers through cell divisions longer than other cells, and they can transform into specialized cells like skin cells. Stem-cell-derived products are used in skin care products to create a protein-signaling cascade to get your cells to shape up and do a better job.
- Stabilizing agents to keep your skin moisturized.

As you begin the Lancer Advanced Anti-Aging Method, you will add one product at a time and start slowly. If you go for a mixed cocktail of all the new treatments to start, your skin will be in for a shock and would react accordingly, turning red and flaky. It could take you anywhere from four to six months to incorporate all the treatments into your routine. Remember: There are no quick fixes with the Lancer Method. Your skin will improve steadily as you provide what it needs to rejuvenate.

A QUICK GUIDE TO ANTI-AGING INGREDIENTS

You will be working your way up to using a number of products that will help to restore your skin. Skin care product manufacturers often spotlight a particular ingredient and invest it with magical, transformative powers. Do not be tricked by their unfounded claims. It is worth your time to know the ingredients to look for on the labels of the products you buy. The products in the list that follows have been scientifically tested and proven to affect the skin positively. There is a whole new category of ingredients that have been labeled "cosmeceuticals," because they have drug-like effects on the skin's structure and functions. These ingredients have proven anti-aging attributes. Some have healing properties for acne, rosacea, and sensitive skin as well. After all, these conditions are all on the same continuum of inflammation.

Glycosaminoglycans

Glycosaminoglycans (GAGs) are the body's natural moisturizers. They hold moisture within skin cells and provide volume, elasticity, and firmness. The most common GAG found in the body is hyaluronic acid.

Keratolytic Agents: AHAs, Glycolic Acid, BHA, Salicylic Acid

These ingredients are exfoliants that remove dead and damaged cells, reducing fine lines, age spots, discoloration, and acne scars. They invigorate, add radiance to the skin, and allow other anti-aging ingredients to penetrate faster, deeper, and more effectively, because they disrupt the stratum corneum. These acids break the bond between the dead cells of the stratum corneum and the skin beneath. It may be helpful to know that retinoids may be deactivated by simultaneous application of AHAs.

Alpha Hydroxy Acids (AHAs) and Glycolic Acid

AHAs are water-soluble. They have a positive effect on sun-damaged skin. AHAs bind moisture and improve collagen production. Glycolic acid is the original AHA used in skin care products. It can irritate and scar darker skins. Introduce AHAs gradually to your regimen, starting once a week. Using a product that contains the AHA mandelic or malic acid may be safer for darker skin ethnicities.

Recommended Glycolic Acid Creams

Luxury:
Lancer Skincare Retexturizing Treatment Cream
Malin & Goetz 10% Glycolic Acid Pads
RéVive Glycolic Renewal Peel

Moderate:
Peter Thomas Roth Glycolic Acid 10% Moisturizer

Cane & Austin Retexturizing Treatment Pads

Affordable:
NeoStrata Face Cream Plus
Aqua Glycolic Face Cream

Beta Hydroxy Acid and Salicylic Acid

Since these exfoliants are fat-soluble, they can penetrate the oil in pores, unclogging them and clearing the debris. Their anti-bacterial and anti-inflammatory properties make them effective with oily skin prone to blackheads, and acne. BHAs also reduce redness from rosacea.

Once Was Quite Enough

A very well-maintained woman in her late fifties wanted to explore better-quality skin care and in-office treatments. She'd had a mini lower neck lift five years earlier and was disappointed with the results. It was painful, she had scarring, and she did not look as great as she'd expected to. Her husband thought the procedure was a waste of money.

She had followed the crowd. So many of her women friends had chosen surgical intervention, and all they talked about was their procedures. So she jumped right in and committed to the mini lift, which she regrets doing to this day.

She came to see me because she wanted to perk things up, to look fresher, but she was not willing even to consider anything invasive. We talked for a while. Agreeing to try better-quality skin care, she was willing to give the Lancer Advanced Anti-Aging Method a chance.

I am glad to see that more and more women are coming to this conclusion about invasive quick fixes. For many of them, once is enough. Rarely do the results meet their expectations, and those are the lucky ones. On top of that disappointment, many feel they threw their money away. Then there are those who have had disastrous results. Scarring, pain, sides of the face not matching, and additional expense to correct problems have made that group say, "Never again!" Almost all of the people I see do not want to return to that arena if they have been there before. They prefer to take care of their skin themselves and to enhance their efforts now and then with non-invasive treatments. With such amazing advances in treatment options, cosmetic, anti-aging surgery will become a thing of the past.

The Takeaway: Skin care combined with non-invasive treatments is the wave of the future.

Anti-Oxidants

Anti-oxidants save cells from environmental damage. As you already know, anti-oxidants turn scavenging free radicals into harmless compounds and stop them from destroying DNA, collagen, and elastin. Topical anti-oxidants supplement the body's innate defense to neutralize free radicals. They boost cell repair, stimulate collagen production, and reduce blotchiness. Although some anti-oxidants multi-task, they are more powerful when they work in packs, because they tackle free radicals in different ways. Here are some specific topical anti-oxidants and what each does.

Vitamin C (L-ascorbic acid)

Known as the workhorse of anti-aging ingredients, vitamin C is the most abundant anti-oxidant in your skin. Not only does it neutralize those age-promoting free radicals that cause inflammation, but vitamin C contributes to the production of new collagen, thickening the skin and reducing fine lines and wrinkles. This powerhouse strengthens the skin barrier by stimulating the production of lipids, which keep the skin from drying out. Vitamin C works synergistically with vitamin E to boost the effectiveness of sunscreen, further protecting the skin from sun damage. At concentrations of 5 percent or higher, vitamin C works to correct hyperpigmentation. Vitamin C enhances the repair process you will already be stimulating with the Lancer Advanced Anti-Aging Method.

Recommended Vitamin C Creams

Luxury:
- Lancer Skincare Advanced C Radiance Cream
- Erno Laszlo Luminous Dual Phase Vitamin C Peel
- Natura Bissé C+C Vitamin Complex
- Sisley-Paris Phyto-Blanc Clearing Essence with Vitamin C

Moderate:
- Kiehl's Clearly Corrective Hydrating Moisture Emulsion
- Dermalogica MAP-15 Regenerator

Affordable:
- Lumene Vitamin C+ Pure Radiance Day Cream SPF 15
- Aveeno Active Naturals Smart Essentials Nighttime Moisture Infusion

---

Vitamin E (Tocophenols, Tocotrienols, Tocophenyl Acetate)

This vitamin, which is fat-soluble, is concentrated mainly in the stratum corneum to absorb the oxidative stress from UV radiation. It protects cell membranes and prevents collagen from being destroyed by UV rays. Vitamin E boosts the skin's natural moisture retention mechanisms. It protects from the formation of age spots and scarring.

Alpha Lipoic Acid

This anti-oxidant is found in every cell of the body. Alpha lipoic acid protects against environmental stressors, including UV radiation, cigarette smoke, auto exhaust, and ozone, all of which can cause oxidative stress. It erases fine lines, diminishes pores, and gives the skin radiance. It is both water- and fat-soluble, which makes it very versatile.

Coenzyme Q10

As you age, your body makes less of the anti-oxidant CoQ10. It has been shown to reduce facial wrinkles, particularly around the eyes. Its anti-aging actions include promoting the proliferation of fibroblasts, which produce collagen and intracellular matrix, and enhancing production of the cells in the epidermal basal membrane.

Selenium

This essential trace mineral has anti-inflammatory and anti-oxidant properties. Selenium helps prevent skin cancer by protecting cell membranes from oxidative deterioration and UV ray damage. This mineral works synergistically with vitamin E.

Retinoids (Retinol, Retinyl Palmitate)

Retinol is a key ingredient for skin renewal. It is a vitamin A derivative that acts on DNA to promote healthy keratinocytes, which results in desired epidermal thickening. Retinol stimulates growth hormones to increase the production of collagen and elastin as it decreases the production of collagenase, the enzyme that eats up collagen. Retinoids sweep away dull, dead cells and speed up cell turnover and repair. The powerful ingredient pumps up circulation in the skin and increases blood vessel formation. And it does not end with that. Retinoids also shrink oil glands and tighten the skin.

Recommended Retinol Creams

Luxury:
Lancer Skincare Regenerative Serum
La Prairie Cellular Power Charge Night
Erno Laszlo Anti Blemish Control
    Treatment

Moderate:
Peter Thomas Roth Retinol Fusion AM
    Moisturizer SPF 30

Kiehl's Powerful-Strength Line-
    Reducing Concentrate

Affordable:
RoC Retinol Correxion products
La Roche-Posay Redermic 0.1% Pure
    Retinol/Retinol Booster Complex

When you first begin to use products containing retinoids, your skin might become scaly. If it does, cut back how often you use it. Your sensitivity to the product should stop in about six to eight weeks. Retinoids can make your skin sensitive to the sun for up to several months. Be certain to use sunscreen when you have added a product containing a retinoid to your skin care routine.

Skin Brighteners

The number one concern of most of my patients is the desire to even out their skin tone. They want to reduce blotchiness and mottled skin and eliminate sun spots. Skin brighteners are often used for pre-procedure conditioning to reduce post-inflammatory hyperpigmentation for patients with an LES of IV or V. Brighteners work by inhibiting the enzyme tyrosinase, which signals the production of melanin in the skin.

Red Algae Extract (Palmaria palmata; *Oligosaccharide)*

This extract from marine algae revitalizes and moisturizes stressed skin by protecting the dermal matrix and stimulating and protecting the epidermal barrier. It fights against redness and uneven skin tone as well.

Phenylethyl Resorcinol

This is a new lightening and brightening ingredient. It's an anti-oxidant that is effective in influencing the formation of pigmentation.

Hydroquinone

This is an effective skin lightener that may or may not have some serious health risks, particularly for people with darker complexions. Since it blocks the production of melanin, the skin's protection from UV rays is diminished, resulting in increased cancer risk. Many darker-skinned women have found that using the substance can whiten the skin long-term, or cause excess discoloration. Hydroquinone is frowned upon in some countries around the world, but not in the United States. When you choose a skin brightener, make certain other brighteners are in the compound and that hydroquinone is not the first ingredient. Hydroquinone can be an irritant, particularly in concentrations of 4 percent or more and when combined with tretinoin.

The beauty industry has been looking for skin lighteners that are as effective.

Alpha-Arbutin

Alpha-arbutin is derived from the leaves of blueberry, mulberry, cranberry, and bearberry bushes. It is a natural source of hydroquinone and has the same melanin-inhibiting properties. It has been found to be a somewhat effective alternative to hydroquinone.

Resveratrol

Resveratrol is a powerful anti-oxidant and anti-inflammatory found in red grape skin that suppresses excess melanin production. You might know it as the "red wine anti-oxidant." That is why you will find grape seed oil in skin care products. It is also found in açaí oil, made from a South American berry. In addition, the spice turmeric is a source of resveratrol. Resveratrol also improves mitochondrial function, the production of energy in the cells.

Recommended Skin Brighteners

Luxury:
Lancer Skincare Fade Serum Intense
Chanel Le Blanc de Chanel
La Prairie White Caviar Illuminating Serum
Kanebo Sensai Silk Brightening Cream SPF 8
Sisley-Paris Phyto-Blanc Intensive Lightening Serum

Moderate:
Clinique Even Better Clinical Dark Spot Corrector

Estée Lauder Idealist Even Skintone Illuminator

Affordable:
La Roche-Posay Mela-D Dark Spots HQ Free, SPF 15
Neutrogena Ageless Intensives Tone Correcting Daily Moisturizer Broad Spectrum SPF 30

Azelaic Acid

Azelaic acid, a component of wheat, barley, rye, and other grains, is used to treat acne. It has proven helpful in treating skin discolorations.

Kojic Acid

This acid is produced by the fermentation of rice in the production of sake. It is a somewhat effective melanin inhibitor. Kojic acid is an unstable ingredient, but kojic dipalmitate, an anti-oxidant, is more stable and used in cosmetics.

Licorice Extract

Produced from the root of the licorice plant, licorice extract is recommended for treating eczema, psoriasis, herpes, and canker sores. Liquiritin, a substance found in licorice, has been found effective in treating melasma, a hyperpigmentation disorder. Manufacturers are beginning to use the extract in cosmetic products.

Peptides

Peptides are short chains of amino acids, the building blocks of proteins. Since they are too big to penetrate the skin barrier, they are engineered in the lab for skin care products and synthesized into different combinations so that they can enter the stratum corneum and affect the functioning of the epidermis and dermis. For example, fatty acids can be added to form lipopeptides, which enhance penetration into the skin.

Peptides were first used topically to heal wounds and reduce the formation of scar tissue, promoting the production of normal skin cells. Peptides are used to regulate the growth rates of skin cells, to limit oxidation, and to create an anti-inflammatory environment—all optimal healing conditions. To counter the effects of aging, your skin needs the same regenerative actions, which is why peptides have made their way into anti-aging products.

Several kinds of peptides are used for skin care:

- Pentapeptides are created when five peptides are linked together. Palmitoyl pentapeptide-3 is a signal peptide that stimulates collagen and elastin production.
- Oligopeptides contain six, seven, or more linked peptide units. Those with seven units can be called heptapeptides. They also stimulate collagen, elastin, and hyaluronic acid production. One common ingredient in beauty products is palmitoyl oligopeptide.
- Copper peptides, the hookup of a peptide with a copper molecule, are carrier peptides that are small enough to travel into the dermis to stimulate collagen growth and boost skin healing. The copper acts as an anti-oxidant.
- Neuropeptides affect neurotransmitters in the skin, relaxing nerve cells and blocking the transmission of signals from nerves to facial muscles. Hexapeptide-48, a nature-derived neuro-calming peptide, is believed to act as a "minor" neurotoxin like Botox to relax wrinkles. More research has to be done to establish the effectiveness of neuropeptides.

Peptide signals to fibroblasts and skin cells contribute significantly to refreshing your skin. A list of the curative actions of peptides will give you a clear picture of why they are an important part of any anti-aging skin care plan:

- Stimulate dermal fibroblasts to produce collagen
- Down-regulate the production of collagenase, the enzyme that eats up collagen
- Stimulate anti-oxidant enzymes
- Enhance matrix proteins
- Regulate wound healing and cell repair
- Speed up skin cell turnover
- Modulate pigmentation
- Produce anti-microbial activity

Peptides help to accomplish all the goals of the Lancer Method.

The Mystique of Stem Cells

A brief history of stem cell use in skin care products will clear up the misconceptions surrounding this ingredient. About twenty years ago, stem cells from human fetuses were harvested and used illegally for spinal cord, cancer, and anti-aging treatments. The use of fetal stem cells was banned in the United States for ethical reasons. The next development involved stem cells harvested from human placentas and amniotic sacs after a live birth. The stem cells were lyophilized, or freeze-dried, and converted to a powder while preserving their original biological properties. After processing, the stem cells are no longer alive. Lyophilizing the living stem cells produces proteins and enzyme derivatives that are bioactive, which is what makes the use of stem cells in treatments and products so effective.

About ten years ago there was a shift, and stem cells began to be derived from sheep placentas and amniotic sacs. The sheep are carefully raised and disease-free. No animals are harmed in harvesting the stem cells. These cell products are close to human stem cell protein. When the animal cells are processed, a protein soup that nourishes human skin is created.

Now plant sources for stem cells are popular. Though you might not think of plants as a potential source for stem cells, even plants have to reproduce. Swiss apple is currently touted as a wholesome, non-controversial source of stem cells, and is used in many popular products. Lancer Skincare products use ocean-based algae, which are rich in proteins, to nourish the skin, along with criste-marine stem cells, from a marine plant native to coastal regions of France, and lilac stem cells.

Stem cells have the power to restore your skin. Here are just a few of the benefits:

- Even skin tone and lighten freckles, dark spots, and uneven pigmentation
- Increase elasticity and reduce sagging
- Hydrate the skin
- Smooth skin, erasing lines and wrinkles
- Reduce the appearance of scars and large pores
- Regulate sebum production
- Enhance the skin's renewal process

Stem cell therapy triggers skin cells to reproduce and to communicate more clearly with each other. Using a firming stem cell cream is an important part of the Lancer Advanced Anti-Aging Method.

Recommended Firming Treatments

Luxury:
Lancer Skincare Lift Serum Intense
AmorePacific Time Response Skin
    Renewal Gel Creme
La Prairie Skin Caviar Liquid Lift
Kanebo Sensai Cellular Performance
    Wrinkle Repair Collagenergy SPF 20

Moderate:
Clarins Extra-Firming Day Wrinkle
    Lifting Cream

Elizabeth Arden Ceramide Plump
    Perfect Ultra Lift and Firm Moisture
    Cream SPF 30

Affordable:
NeoStrata Skin Active Cellular
    Restoration
Nivea Body Skin Firming Moisturizer
    Q10 Plus with Advanced Q10
Physicians Formula Rx 132 Expression
    Line Freeze Serum

Stabilizing Agents

The strength of the stratum corneum is derived from lipids, proteins, and water. Ceramides constitute half the cornified layer's lipid or fat content. The lipids between skin cells seal them together. Ceramides are critical components of the skin barrier that keeps moisture in and pathogens out. These fats keep your skin healthy and vibrant. The ceramide content in your skin decreases with sun damage. The following ingredients boost ceramide levels and free fatty acid levels in skin:

Niacinamide (B₃)

Niacinamide is a water-soluble vitamin that increases ceramide levels, which prevents the skin from losing water by stimulating circulation in the dermis through vasodilation. This vitamin decreases lines and wrinkles by increasing dermal protein and collagen production. It is gaining a reputation for lightening skin discoloration and reducing acne. Niacinamide is known to reduce the yellowing of skin, which results from the glycation of proteins that comes with aging. As an anti-oxidant, it improves epidermal barrier function and quiets inflammation.

Hyaluronic Acid

This is a sugar produced by the body to keep tissues cushioned and lubricated. It's found in the skin, joint fluid, and connective tissue. Hyaluronic acid levels decrease over time with aging, smoking, and unhealthy eating habits. Hyaluronic acid absorbs water and plumps up skin. When used as an ingredient in moisturizers, it helps skin to repair and regenerate in response to dryness, environmental stresses, or irritation. Hyaluronic acid is effective when combined with vitamin C to smooth skin.

Linoleic Acids and Phospholipids

These free fatty acids function to replenish the intercellular matrix. They are good communicators that increase the skin's own anti-oxidant nature. They prevent anti-oxidant enzyme depletion and DNA degradation.

Recommended Night Creams

Luxury:
  Lancer Skincare Intensive Night
    Treatment
  Erno Laszlo Firmarine Night Cream
  Sisley-Paris Intensive Night Cream

Moderate:
  Elizabeth Arden Plump Perfect Ultra
    All Night Repair and Moisture
    Cream
  Dermalogica Overnight Repair Serum

  Estée Lauder Advanced Time Zone
    Night Age Reversing Wrinkle/Line
    Creme

Affordable:
  Aveeno Active Naturals Skin Relief
    Overnight Cream, Intense Moisture
  Neutrogena Naturals Multi-Vitamin
    Nourishing Night Cream
  RoC Multi Correxion Lift Anti-Gravity
    Night Cream

Botanicals

Today more than seventy natural ingredients from plants have been used in skin care products. Just a few top ingredients will be covered here.

Caffeine

Caffeine used as a topical ingredient is an anti-oxidant that can inhibit the growth of skin cancer. It has the power to reduce wrinkles, especially crow's-feet.

Isoflavones

Derived from soy, isoflavones are plant estrogens that mimic some of estrogen's effects on the skin. Phytoestrogens couple with estrogen receptors, which are densest in the granular layer. They keep the skin from thinning and correct dryness and loss of elasticity. They are anti-oxidants that combat free radicals and increase the production of collagen and hyaluronic acid.

Green Tea

This has anti-oxidant and anti-inflammatory properties. The anti-aging benefits of green tea are attributed to polyphenols, a type of flavonoids found in plants. Early studies have shown that green tea can reduce sun damage, protect skin from cancer, and decrease collagen breakdown. The polyphenols are thought to influence biochemical pathways that lead to cell regeneration.

Marula Oil

This oil comes from the fruit of the marula tree from South Africa, where it is used as a moisturizer. A hydrating ingredient, it contains high levels of omega fatty acids and anti-oxidants. Marula oil softens the skin and balances moisture levels.

Since there is such high demand for the next new wonder ingredient, research for anti-aging products is at a fever pitch. Though the beauty trap has no problem exaggerating the effects of the latest "breakthrough" in skin care, ingredients that are authentically effective are being discovered all the time. The formulations for skin care products are much more sophisticated than they were just two years ago, and topicals will only continue to improve.

The Lancer Advanced Anti-Aging Method

This list includes all the elements of the advanced regimen. Your skin has already acclimated to the polish, cleanse, nourish steps of the Lancer Method now that you have been doing it for several months. Beginning the Lancer Advanced Method will take your skin to the next level of rejuvenation—if you need it. It could take you up to six months to do the full advanced anti-aging regimen, because you have to introduce new treatments gradually. This list indicates the order in which the products should be used in the morning and at night. You can increase the penetration of the products by spraying your face lightly with springwater before applying each. Doing this is like using low-calorie mayonnaise on a sandwich to bind the layers of ingredients.

A.M.

Cleanse
Treat:
Glycolic acid cream
Eye cream
Nourish
Sunscreen SPF 30

P.M.

Polish
Cleanse
Treat:
Vitamin C cream
Firming serum
Night cream
Skin brightening serum
Eye cream
Nourish

HOW TO EASE INTO THE LANCER ADVANCED ANTI-AGING METHOD

To be successful with the Lancer Advanced Anti-Aging Method, you have to grow to understand your skin, which changes all the time and will respond to treatments differently from day to day. The weather, your mood, the varying levels of stress in your life, how much you had to drink at that party, and countless other factors affect your metabolism and the amount of oxygen that circulates to your skin. As you age, your metabolism slows—and so does oxygen transport, which fuels regeneration. The state of your skin is dynamic, not static. That is why the Lancer Method works. If the Lancer Method is going to stimulate biochemical changes in your skin, it has to react. You will make the connection among lifestyle and other factors, treatments, and the condition of your skin in time with close observation.

Taking the Lancer Method to the fine-tuned stage is a flexible, individualized process. By observing how your skin responds to new treatments, you can approach the fine-tuned Lancer Method presented in this and the next three chapters as an artist mixes a palette. It is up to you to decide when to increase the number of times a week that you use a product and when your skin is ready for layering in another treatment.

At first, some products might sting slightly, and your face might flush. If the reaction is intense and your skin becomes dry, red, and scaly, use the product only once a week until your skin drinks it in without protest. If you have a moderate reaction, do not use the product every day. Instead, use it every other day until your skin no longer reacts. You have to make a judgment about whether your skin is ready for the next step. One thing you can count on—your skin will let you know when it is not happy. Observe it closely and slow down if your skin becomes irritated in any way. You do not have to rush. The products that you are already using will be doing their work to make your skin look and behave younger. This process could take two, four, or six months, depending on your skin.

I suggest that you add a new product each week to your basic polish-cleanse-nourish-sunscreen regimen until you are doing the full Lancer Advanced Method. This is the order I recommend to introduce new products:

Week 1: Eye cream a.m./p.m.
Week 2: Vitamin C cream p.m.
Week 3: Glycolic acid cream a.m.
Week 4: Retinol cream p.m.
Week 5: Firming treatment p.m.
Week 6: Night cream p.m.
Week 7: Brightening serum p.m.

From the basic program, you will already be cleansing and nourishing in the morning and at night, using sunblock in the morning and polishing at night. Start slowly when you introduce a new product. Layer the products, applying them one at a time. There is no need to wait between applications. Lancer Skincare products have interlocking chemistry. One product enhances the effectiveness of the others. If you are pressed for time, you can mix the various treatment creams in the palm of your hand and do a single application. Of course, eye cream will have to be applied separately. Do not mix in other brands, which may have conflicting chemistry and ingredients that could interfere with the method.

Use a product only one day the first week you try it, then add a day each consecutive week. According to this schedule, you will be using all the products every day by the twelfth week, at three months. Keep in mind, everyone has a unique metabolism. It might take you more or less time to introduce all the products. Incorporating new products into your routine in this way will help you to identify the source of any sensitivity or problem. If your skin reacts to a product you have just introduced, you should build up more slowly, maybe using that product just once a week for a month.

A Program for Introducing New Products

PRODUCT	WEEK 1	WEEK 2	WEEK 3	WEEK 4	WEEK 5	WEEK 6	WEEK 7	WEEK 8	WEEK 9	WEEK 10	WEEK 11	WEEK 12	WEEK 13
A.M.													
Cleanse	X	X	X	X	X	X	X	X	X	X	X		
Glycolic acid			1 DAY	2	3	4	5	6	7				
Eye cream	1 DAY	2	3	4	5	6	7						
Nourish	X	X	X	X	X	X	X	X	X	X	X		
Sunblock SPF 30	X	X	X	X	X	X	X	X	X	X	X		
P.M.													
Polish	X	X	X	X	X	X	X	X	X	X	X		
Cleanse	X	X	X	X	X	X	X	X	X	X	X		
Vitamin C cream		1 DAY	2.	3	4	5	6	7					
Retinol cream				1 DAY	2	3	4	5	6	7			
Firming treatment					1 DAY	2	3	4	5	6	7		
Night cream						1 Day	2	3	4	5	6	7	
Brightening serum							1 Day	2	3	4	5	6	7
Eye cream	1 DAY	2	3	4	5	6	7						
Nourish	X	X	X	X	X	X	X	X	X	X	X		

If this regimen seems daunting to you, I assure you that once you get the hang of it, the routine will become automatic. When you are in a big hurry, you can take a shortcut, as I noted above. Instead of applying each product one by one, take a dab of the products you are using and combine them in your hand, mix them with a fingertip, and apply all of them together. Layering the products is more effective, but it is better to apply them than to skip treating your skin.

You do not have to follow this routine to the letter. You might want to take your time adding new products. After reading the descriptions of the anti-aging products in this chapter, you might not feel you need a particular anti-aging product. The cleanse-polish-nourish-sunscreen steps are a must. After that, it is up to you. At some point, you might feel as if you have taken your skin as far as it can go with the products you are using and decide to try something new to see if there are even more improvements. Once you have dealt with some signs of aging, others might become more noticeable.

If you want to focus on specific skin issues, here are some suggestions for the products to use:

- **Enhanced tone balance regimen:** Glycolic acid cream and skin brightener
- **Enhanced lift and radiance regimen:** Vitamin C cream and brightening serum
- **Enhanced texture corrector regimen:** Glycolic acid cream and sunscreen
- **Enhanced eye-area care regimen:** Eye cream and firming serum
- **Enhanced lifting and smoothing regimen:** Firming serum and night cream

Application

As with the basic Lancer Anti-Aging Method, I recommend doing the polish and cleanse steps in the shower, because thirty seconds of steam will moisten your skin well so that you can get a deep cleanse. At this point, you should be expert with the polish-cleanse-nourish basic program. The first new treatment you will be adding is an eye-brightening cream. Since the early signs of aging show around the eyes where the skin is thin and delicate, fine wrinkles and dark circles are of great concern to patients of all ages. It is never too soon to begin treatment for this vulnerable area. Using well-formulated products can help reduce fine lines

Recommended Eye Creams

Luxury:

Lancer Skincare Eye Contour Lifting Cream

Chanel Sublimage La Crème Yeux

AmorePacific Moisture Bound Intensive Vitalizing Eye Complex

La Mer The Eye Concentrate

Aesop Parsley Seed Anti-Oxidant Eye Cream (sensitive)

Jurlique Herbal Recovery Eye Cream (sensitive)

Moderate:

Dermalogica Age Reversal Eye Complex

Kiehl's Line-Reducing Eye-Brightening Concentrate

Clinique All About Eyes

Clarins Super Restorative Total Eye Concentrate (sensitive)

Valmont Expression Line Reducer Eye Factor

Affordable:

RoC Retinol Correxion Eye Cream

L'Oréal Paris Revitalift Triple Power Eye Treatment

Neutrogena Rapid Wrinkle Repair Eye Cream

Aveeno Positively Ageless Lifting & Firming Eye Cream

La Roche-Posay Substiane (+) Eyes

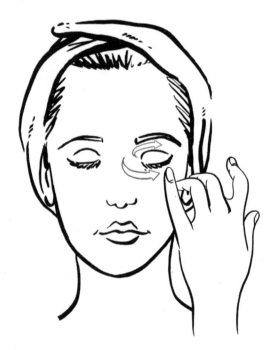

and wrinkles, reduce puffiness, and fade dark pigmentation under the eyes.

Eye cream is best applied with your pinkie. With your eye closed, start with your lower lid. From the bridge of your nose outward, dab the eye cream along the line of the lower bone of your eye socket to where it meets the upper bone in the outer corner of your eye. Apply little dabs on your upper lid from the bridge of your nose and follow the bone of your upper eye socket under your eyebrow outward to the corner. The cream will be absorbed by the skin and affect the entire area.

This chapter has given you an intensive program to make your skin look healthy and younger. The Lancer Advanced Anti-Aging Method will delay aging if you are trying to preserve your skin as it

Adult Training Wheels

A yoga teacher in her early sixties had an appointment with our permanent makeup artist to have work done on her eyebrows. She did not wear makeup, and her eyebrows were indistinct. She thought her faded eyebrows made her look too vague. She was at the office for a touch-up.

This woman, a vegan, was five foot seven and weighed 105 pounds. She looked sallow and, to my eye, could have used some animal protein. The permanent makeup artist advised her that she should do more to take care of her skin. I was called in. As usual, I handed her a mirror and a Q-tip and asked her if anything bothered her about her skin. All she saw was some brown spots.

In addition to being sallow, her face was covered with fine lines, she had the beginnings of jowls, and her skin was papery. She clearly was a case of low-density collagen, because of her genetics, diet, and sun exposure. Though extrinsic and intrinsic aging were visible on her face, she was reluctant to do anything about it. She had seen her friends do drastic things and was horrified by the results. She was stuck in her thinking, a purist, and not inclined to try cosmetic improvement of any sort. But at-home skin care did not sound too threatening. She began to do the basic Lancer Method.

She called to let us know that she felt good and had experienced no irritation or sensitivity. She gained confidence as her skin became more vibrant. Not wanting to alarm her, we took infinite care when introducing new products to her skin care routine. Her negativity and reluctance evaporated. She is doing the full Lancer Advanced Anti-Aging Method now, and her skin has responded beautifully.

The Takeaway: It is never too late to improve your skin, especially if you have never taken special care of it. Patient confidence and trust are great helps.

is now and to prevent premature damage. The Lancer Method will increase your skin's oxygen level and stimulate cell turnover for fresher, glowing skin. Investing the time and effort now to maintain your skin's radiance and smoothness will keep you from wanting extreme procedures later. If you are coming late to the party, you can correct damage before it is beyond fixing if you make the Lancer Advanced Anti-Aging Method a way of life. The next three chapters deal with conditions that require special attention: acne, rosacea, and sensitive skin. Nearly 85 percent of all Americans have had acne in their lives. At any given time, the number of people in the United States with acne is about sixty million. Rosacea affects fourteen million. The results of one survey found that 45 percent of the participants claimed to have sensitive skin. Judging from my practice, the number is actually higher.

These conditions have a devastating effect on self-esteem and afflict people of all ages and every skin color. I have customized the Lancer Method to treat these conditions with excellent results. If you have not had any of these problems to date, that does not mean you will not develop any of them in the future. They can affect you at any point in life. If you have acne- or rosacea-prone skin or reactive, sensitive skin, read on. One of the next three chapters is for you.

7

The Lancer Anti-Aging Method for Acne-Prone Skin

If you are lucky, you might wonder why an anti-aging book has a chapter on acne. You might assume that pimples are a thing of the past, a bad memory from adolescence. The fact is that 30 percent of women and 20 percent of men from the ages of twenty to sixty are troubled by acne breakouts. Though teenage boys have more acne scarring than girls, women are more likely than men to have adult acne.

Though a bad case of acne can have a negative impact on the self-esteem of an already self-conscious teenager, a breakout or even a single pimple can be a major source of distress and embarrassment for an adult. Adolescent acne lesions tend to appear on the upper half of the face. Adult acne is usually concentrated in the central part of the face and along the jawline. Adults get isolated pimples, but they are whoppers. Teenage breakouts are mostly superficial. In contrast, acne lesions in adults are deep under the skin and become cystic. Adult skin can develop enlarged pores and ruddiness along with acne blemishes.

A Cool, Calm, and Collected Leader

Among my patients is an international political figure in his sixties, who finds himself in Los Angeles often. He came to consult with me because he was very concerned about his appearance. He travels continually, and his complexion was showing signs of accumulated abuse. His skin had become greasy and blemished. He thought his appearance could send the wrong message.

He frequently attended high-stakes diplomatic and business meetings with other political and industrial leaders. He wanted his looks to communicate to the powerful people in attendance that he was unflappable and in control. He confided in me that he had advisers on his team trained to read the faces of his opponents. Everyone did, he assured me. He was convinced that his red, oily, broken-out skin made him look nervous and weak.

I put him on my blemish protocol and monitored his diet, being certain that he ate more estrogenic foods. You will read why later in this chapter. His skin improved in time, and his confidence was restored.

The Takeaway: The condition of your skin can telegraph your internal state to others.

For some, acne has been a constant state since their teenage years. Others experience a recurrence after years of clear skin. Breakouts can occur for the first time during pregnancy, perimenopause, menopause, or times of extreme stress. Many women and men are dealing with acne at the same time they are trying to combat the effects of aging on their skin. Of the sixty million Americans who have acne, twenty million have it severely enough to cause scars.

It might surprise you to know that acne and aging are on the same spectrum. The mechanisms and physical processes that cause your skin to age are also responsible for acne. Changes in the balance of the epidermis create the conditions that result in clogged pores, the root of this common skin disorder. Acne is associated with abnormalities in epidermal barrier functions. The Lancer Method works to heal acne in the same way it revitalizes and restores aging skin. Before we get to the cure, we have to understand the problem.

THE MAKING OF A PIMPLE

Acne is a disorder of the pilosebaceous unit or PSU. This unit consists of sebaceous or oil glands connected to a follicle that may or may not produce a shaft of hair. For every hair on your body, there is a corresponding skin pore, but not every pore houses a hair. Pores are found everywhere except the palms, soles of the feet, lower lip, and parts of the genital area. PSUs are densest on the face, neck, chest, back, and shoulders. That is where the skin disruptions of acne occur.

When canals and pores become plugged with oil and dead skin cells, acne develops. A pimple forms when the sebaceous glands produce too much sebum. The severity of acne corresponds to the amount of oil produced. Normally, sebum keeps skin and hair moisturized. The oily skin of adolescence results from the hormone surge typical of that period of life, which leads to excessive amounts of sebum. After the age of twenty, sebum production begins to decrease. Hormonal imbalance caused by the menstrual cycle, pregnancy, perimenopause, and menopause leads to the reduction of estrogen and the relative increase of male hormones in women. That is why more women experience adult-onset acne. The proportion of male hormones becomes higher, creating an excess of sebum that leads to acne for some people.

Microcomedone

- The sebum combines with keratinocytes within the canal and cells ready to be sloughed off from the stratum corneum. The corneocytes become too sticky to shed and accumulate in the pores.
- The mix of dead cells and oil can form a plug in the canal. As the material builds up, a bottleneck is formed, called a microcomedone, a precursor to an acne lesion that is not yet visible. Microcomedones can develop into full-blown comedones that can be inflamed or not.

Inflammatory Immune Response

- *P. acnes* (*Propionibacterium acnes*) bacteria that normally live on the skin feed on the mixture of sebum and dead skin cells, thrive, and can set off an inflammatory immune response, drawing white blood cells to fight the bacteria.

Bursting of Follicle

- When the plugged follicle canal can no longer hold its contents, the pus bursts and spills into the dermis, resulting in a spreading inflammation and more tissue destruction.

Comedones

Whitehead or Closed Comedone

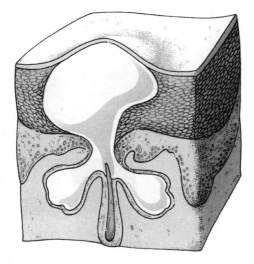

Blackhead or Open Comedone

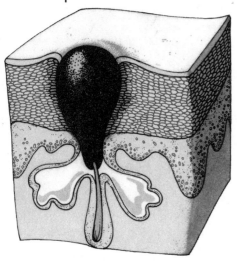

A microcomedone can evolve into a number of different lesions that represent the stages of acne. Whiteheads and blackheads are comedones that are not inflamed.

When the pore becomes clogged and bloated with the oil, dead skin cell, and bacteria mixture that stays beneath the skin, a whitehead or closed comedone forms. The area becomes a slightly raised bump on the skin.

With an open comedone, the mixture is exposed to air at the skin's surface through an open pore, and the plug darkens. The pores become black spots or blackheads.

Inflammatory Papule

If bacteria enter the picture, acne lesions become inflamed. The simplest form is called a papule, which is a small pink bump on the skin that is tender. The sebum-corneocyte mix builds up pressure on the cells surrounding the pore. Enough pressure will rupture the sides of the pore; the sebaceous material will leak into the surrounding skin, which gets infected when the *P. acnes* bacteria are released. The small red bump that appears is an inflammatory papule.

Pustule

An acne pustule, commonly known as a pimple, is the next stage. White blood cells have appeared at the site to fight off the *P. acnes* infection. White blood cells pile up and create pus at the tip of the bump, which is red at the base. Pustules are often mistaken for whiteheads for this reason.

Nodule

A more troublesome lesion is the nodule, a large, painful, solid lesion that is lodged deep within the skin like a boil at the level of the dermis. Nodules cause serious scarring.

Cyst

Finally, inflamed, pus-filled cysts can form deep in the skin. Cysts are painful and also lead to scarring.

If you want to stop acne from intensifying and doing serious damage to your skin, you need to consult a

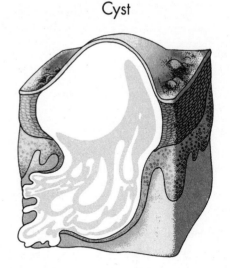

Cyst

The Six Types of Acne

Acne takes many forms, and here they are:

Acne vulgaris is the most common form of acne and the source of everyday breakouts, blackheads, whiteheads, and pimples of varying degrees of severity. This type of acne can be non-inflammatory or inflammatory cystic.

Acne rosacea is like acne vulgaris and is the most common form of acne after vulgaris. This form of acne is distinguished by a red rash that covers the nose, cheeks, forehead, and chin. People confuse this form of acne with rosacea. In fact, they are different disorders. One distinguishing characteristic is that rosacea usually does not produce whiteheads and blackheads. *Rosacea* describes many other skin presentations, which the following chapter will cover.

Acne conglobata is the most severe acne. With this form of acne, large lesions are interconnected across the face and body and accompanied by an abundance of big blackheads. This form of acne leaves serious scars.

Acne fulminans occurs suddenly. It is accompanied by fever and aching joints. It often develops after unsuccessful treatment for acne conglobata.

Pyoderma faciale consists of large nodules and pustules that are very damaging. Like acne fulminans, this type of acne appears suddenly. It appears on the faces of women and men between the ages of twenty and forty. Typically, this condition has swings in activity with more or less severity.

Gram-negative folliculitis, an uncommon condition of pustules and cysts, may be caused by long-term use of antibiotics, particularly tetracycline, for the treatment of acne vulgaris.

A board-certified dermatologist can identify what type of acne is troubling your skin and the best way to treat it.

dermatologist. Over-the-counter remedies might help the occasional breakout, but you need the help of a board-certified dermatologist to avoid scarring and to stop acne's progress.

WHAT IS BEHIND ADULT ACNE FLARE-UPS

Genetics

Whether or not you develop acne largely depends on your genes. Though being acne-prone is an inherited trait, the rising statistics indicate that the cause obviously goes beyond genetics. Lifestyle has a lot to do with it.

Hormones

An overproduction of androgens, or a change in the overall hormone balance in women and men, can cause breakouts. Large amounts of testosterone overstimulate the sebaceous glands, which produce an excess of sebum. During puberty, that hormonal surge causes real problems for male and female skin. As males mature, there is less fluctuation in their hormones than those of the opposite sex.

Females have a monthly cycle of shifting hormone levels. The premenstrual time is a red-hot flare-up zone, because androgens and oil production are high. Androgen-based birth control pills can cause increased oiliness and consequent breakouts. Hormonal fluctuations during pregnancy can also wreak havoc on a woman's skin, resulting in pregnancy acne. The decrease of estrogen with age during perimenopause and menopause reduces the protective function of the female hormones, estrogen in particular. The balance shifts, and androgens have a more powerful effect, resulting in increased oiliness and breakouts.

Stress

Stress makes your skin more sensitive and reactive. It is a leading aggravating factor in acne flare-ups. In general, the body's ability to resist infection is lowered by stress. Stress interrupts the healing process, causing new lesions to form and the breakdown of lesions that had begun to heal. Stress exacerbates any disease by setting an inflammatory cascade into motion. A chronically inflamed body is the ideal environment for the development of acne lesions. When you are stressed, your body produces cortisol and other stress hormones that trigger the production of more oil in your skin. Sudden stress can turn a non-inflammatory lesion into a painful nodule in less than twenty-four hours.

Diet and Acne

The role food plays in the formation of acne is surrounded by controversy. In the past, chocolate, french fries, other fried foods, and sweets were the suspected culprits. Then the thinking changed, and the link between diet and acne was treated as a myth. Now research is taking a broader view of the relationship between diet and acne flare-ups. With the rise in the incidence of acne in the United States, scientists have been studying the impact of the modern Western diet on the skin. They have found an association between obesity and acne. The consumption of dairy products, refined sugar, salt, and foods high on the glycemic index has been found to promote and aggravate acne.

Studies have found that obese people have higher levels of testosterone than people with a normal body mass index (BMI). That alone is enough to stimulate the overproduction of oils that can clog pores. Cow's milk may contain steroid hormones and other components that precipitate a hormonal cascade, overstimulating the pilosebaceous unit described earlier. Processed food, so prevalent in the Western diet, is packed with refined sugar and salt. If you study the labels of processed foods, you will see sucrose, high fructose corn syrup, and salt close to the top of the list. Highly processed food is broken down quickly and converted to glucose, which causes spikes in blood sugar levels. High levels of glucose in the blood trigger the production of more insulin, which leads to inflammation and increased androgen levels. A high-carbohydrate diet can make you acne-prone.

If you reduce your consumption of simple carbohydrates, you will reduce acne symptoms. If you stay away from white foods—potatoes, white bread, white pasta, cakes, cookies, rice—and processed foods and refined sugars, you will reduce acne symptoms. Replace processed foods with whole foods that are high-fiber sources of carbohydrates, such as nuts, vegetables, beans, and fruits. Eat small meals and snacks often during the day to keep your blood sugar level stable. This will improve your acne while fighting aging. Chapter 11 will go more deeply into the right way to eat to look young and feel great, including foods that will stimulate estrogen production.

Medications and Drugs

Certain medications and drugs are known to aggravate acne conditions or cause them. Corticosteroids, mood elevators, anti-anxiety drugs, anti-depressants, certain cold and flu medications, recreational drugs, and DHEA can cause acne breakouts. Discuss the medications you are taking with your dermatologist.

Grooming Products

A major contributing factor for breakouts involves the products you use on your skin and hair. Many cosmetic products—shampoo, conditioner, soap, makeup—are comedogenic, meaning they are acne causing. There is even a form of acne

For Some Patients, a Pimple Is the End of the World

My schedule in the office is frenetic, but we leave some time for walk-in emergencies every day. Whether it is a CEO who has to speak at a shareholders' meeting or a bride two days before her wedding, I see people so thrown by acne flare-ups that their self-confidence is completely undermined. They need immediate attention. People want to look their best for important events. That is when flare-ups are almost sure to happen. I had one such emergency session just the other day.

A patient of many years came to the office a few hours before she had to catch a flight to New York. She was going to appear on one of the big morning TV shows early the next day. She was distressed to find what she considered a disfiguring blemish on the tip of her nose, which no amount of makeup could hide. The good news is that a cyst can be neutralized in two or three hours.

I softened the cyst by applying a warm compress first. I found the exact origin, the affected pore opening, with a 10X magnifying glass. I put an extremely fine, 32-gauge micro-needle directly into the pore. I pierced the skin at the base of the bump with another needle. Then I flushed out the pimple by shooting a syringe filled with a tablespoon of salt water into the pore. The gunk drained through the hole at the top like a volcano. After more warm compresses, I used ice to flatten the bump and make the redness go down.

My patient flew to New York and looked great on TV the next morning.

The Takeaway: Take preemptive action and schedule an appointment with a dermatologist six weeks before an important event. Be sure to make any follow-up visits suggested.

popularly called pomade acne that is caused by hair products that seep into the forehead and trap bacteria in the hair ducts. Your hairstyle can cause or aggravate acne. For example, wearing bangs puts hair care products in direct contact with your skin. If you use products with spray applicators, the chemicals wind up on your face as well as your hair. It is best to keep products away from your hairline and to rinse your face to remove any styling product that remains on your face.

If you change your skin care products or add a new one, you are challenging your skin with new active ingredients, preservatives, and other additives. Your skin can react and break out. Introducing too many new acne products at once can cause blemishes. You should add new products to your regimen gradually, one or two at a time, and give your skin enough time to adjust. About four to six weeks is average.

Even products that are labeled non-comedogenic, water-based, or oil-free might still have irritating ingredients. You will find recommendations for skin care products for blemished skin later in the chapter.

EVERYDAY ACNE TRIGGERS

Genetics, hormones, stress, diet, medications, and cosmetic products constitute the big picture when it comes to the causes of acne, but there are myriad things that can negatively affect acne-prone skin. Making some small adjustments in your life and raising your awareness of situations that can bring on breakouts will help you to keep your skin clear and flawless. Sweat, dirt, and bacteria are major causes of breakouts, so limiting your skin's exposure to these elements is a great place to start.

Here are a few ways to protect your skin from breakouts:

- Do not mess with pimples and blemishes yourself! This can spread bacteria and make the problem worse, or cause scarring.
- Change your pillowcase every few nights to avoid trapped bacteria.
- Avoid the use of fabric softeners on your towels and sheets—they can clog pores and cause irritation.
- Limiting your caffeine intake will reduce breakout-causing inflammation in the skin.

Facial Hair Removal

Waxing, tweezing, depilatories, and laser removal can make skin tissues swell, sending bacteria and skin cells deeper into the pore and follicle shaft. You might be trading facial hair for bumpy skin that itches. Use 1 percent hydrocortisone before and after you defuzz.

Telephone Acne

The surfaces of cell phones and phones in general collect bacteria. The warmth and moisture from your mouth create a perfect environment for bacteria to thrive. Phones are held close to your face and can cause friction acne. It is a good idea to clean your phones with an alcohol wipe or hand sanitizer daily. While you are at it, clean your eyeglasses and sunglasses.

Do Not Wear Makeup at the Gym or When You Are Sweating and Other Workout Tips

Makeup will block your pores and prevent elimination of toxins. It will also suffocate your skin. Wear wicking fabrics for a hard workout. Sweating in tight clothing can lead to excessive oil production and cause acne on your chest and back. Skin swells from freshly oxygenated blood sent to feed working muscles. Perspiration produces acids and salts to cool the body. Combined with the swelling, this is a perfect formula for skin irritation and dryness. Sports glasses, helmets, hats, and headbands should be cleaned well and often if you want to avoid breakouts.

Be Mindful of the Stresses of Travel

Aside from the ordeal of security checks, catching trains and planes, and traffic, the change in your environment created by traveling can affect your skin. If you are going to a tropical climate, heat and humidity can cause acne flare-ups. You sweat to cool off your body, and the acids and salts in perspiration can dry your skin and increase inflammation. If you are traveling to a place that is frigid, cold and ice cause your skin to get thinner. That can be a good thing if you have lesions.

> Extra tip: Before applying topical treatments for acne, you might try icing your face with an ice cube. Just as you ice a sprained ankle to reduce swelling, lesions will shrink in size in the cold. Extreme cold can be drying and is not the answer.

When you are traveling, wash your face with bottled water, because your skin may react to different minerals in the tap water. Avoid using hotel soaps, shampoos, and conditioners, because introducing new products can cause your skin to react.

Pick the Right Non-Irritating Sunscreen for Your Skin

The chemical agents that protect your skin from harmful UV rays either are absorbed by your skin or rest on the skin's surface to create a sun shield. The physical agents that stay on the surface can be bad for acne-prone skin. The ingredients zinc oxide and titanium oxide may sit on the surface and cause sweating that becomes irritating. Use products with avobenzone, oxybenzone, methoxycinnamate, or octocrylene in combination with physical blocks.

Limit Your Caffeine Intake

Drinking coffee or highly caffeinated beverages launches your body into a stressed-out state. What you perceive as energy is created by the fight-or-flight hormones that kick in and create inflammation. To keep your energy high, switch to a diet rich in complex carbohydrates.

THE LANCER METHOD TO THE RESCUE

The basic three-step Lancer Method—polish, cleanse, and nourish—works wonders for acne-prone skin. You will have to use products created specifically for blemished skin. They are formulated to be gentle and non-irritating and to neutralize the bacteria that cause inflammatory acne. You should not use the same products teenagers use. Those products are designed to reduce extreme oiliness. Older skin can be dry and still have acne breakouts. If your skin gets too dry, you will exacerbate acne lesions.

The fine-tuned Lancer Method for skin with problems will require some judgments from you. You will have to observe how your skin behaves and respond accordingly when introducing new products to your regimen. You want to prevent your skin from becoming seriously inflamed and to calm it if it is. For example, if your skin is oily, large-pored, and inflamed, you will want to ease into the three steps. You do not want to risk irritating your skin more. I suggest that you polish just once every other evening the first week and then every evening, five days a week. When your skin is used to that, polish every night. Then repeat introducing the polish step in the morning, so that you will eventually be exfoliating gently twice a day. If your skin gets red, irritated, and dried, cut back on the polishing. You have to judge how much your skin can benefit from this polishing to reach maintenance.

Active Ingredients in Acne Treatment Products

You should be familiar with the five ingredients that you will find in most acne products:

- **Benzoyl peroxide** is used in over-the-counter and prescription products for acne. Benzoyl peroxide dries up excess oil, kills bacteria by flooding them with oxygen, and mildly exfoliates. It can soften up plugs in a couple of weeks and keep more from forming. It is available in strengths from 2.5 to 10 percent. Unless your skin is extremely oily, you should use the lowest strength for adult acne; otherwise, it can cause dryness, scaling, redness, burning, and stinging. Available in gels, lotions, and pads, benzoyl peroxide is sold under various brand names. For older skin, I recommend using mild formulated products that contain this effective blemish fighter. You do not want to dry out your skin. Use it carefully, because it can bleach clothing and hair.
- **Salicylic acid** prevents the pores from clogging by gently increasing cell shedding inside the skin pores. When applied, it can sting and cause irritation. Over-the-counter acne products are available in strengths of 0.5 to 2 percent. Brand names change. Look at the label. Some products are better suited to younger skin.
- Two **alpha hydroxy acids** will appear on the labels of over-the-counter acne products: **glycolic acid** and **lactic acid**. Not only do they remove dead skin cells and help to reduce inflammation, but they also stimulate the growth of new, smooth skin that reduces the appearance of acne scars.
- **Sulfur** is combined with other ingredients, like salicylic acid, benzoyl peroxide, or resorcinol. It works to remove pore-clogging dead skin cells and excess oil. Sulfur may have an unpleasant odor, which is unmistakable, but it can be masked.

These ingredients can irritate the skin initially. It can take up to four weeks before the skin improves.

The Lancer Anti-Acne Method

You will gradually work your way to this schedule. Take it slow. Start by polishing once a week at night. Then polish every other night. Give your skin time to adjust to your new routine before polishing twice a day every day.

A.M.

Exfoliator with salicylic acid
Cleanser for oily or acneic skin
Glycolic acid cream
Oil-free anti-aging face moisturizer

P.M.

Blemish polish
Blemish cleanser
Blemish nourisher
Vitamin C cream
Firming serum
Night cream

Polish for Blemished Skin

Exfoliating is especially important for blemished skin. Acne lesions form when pores are blocked by a plug composed of dead skin cells mixed with sebum. Bacteria can feed on the mixture, and your skin becomes inflamed. Keeping those pores open and exfoliating the dead cell buildup will prevent acne. Sloughing off dead skin cells from the surface of your skin will keep them from blocking pores and preventing the flow of sebum to the skin's surface, where it moisturizes and makes the skin look fresh. Polishing also brings oxygen to the skin, increasing metabolism, which speeds up blemish healing.

If you have inflammatory acne and large pores when you begin using the Lancer Anti-Aging Method for Acne-Prone Skin, ease into it. Polish only one night the first week. Work your way up until you are polishing morning and night. You have to be very gentle if you have acne lesions. You do not want them to burst under the skin and infect surrounding areas.

For blemished skin, you have to find an exfoliant with larger, spherical buffing particles without rough edges to avoid irritating your skin further. If possible, try to sample an exfoliator before buying to be certain that the product is gentle enough for your sensitive skin.

Recommended Exfoliators for Blemished Skin

Look for an exfoliator containing salicylic acid.

Luxury:

Lancer Skincare The Method: Polish Blemish Control

Erno Laszlo Anti Blemish Beta Wash

Sisley-Paris Buff and Wash Botanical Facial Gel Cleanser

Omorovicza Gentle Buffing Cleanser

Moderate:

Bliss Pore Perfecting Facial Polish

Clinique Exfoliating Scrub

First Aid Beauty Facial Radiance Polish

Ahava Facial Mud Exfoliator

Affordable:

L'Oréal Paris Go 360° Clean Deep Exfoliating Scrub

Aveeno Positively Radiant Skin Brightening Daily Scrub

Clearasil Stayclear Daily Facial Scrub

Boots No7 Total Renewal Micro-dermabrasion Exfoliator

Recommended Cleansers for Blemished Skin

Cleanser for blemished skin should have ingredients like salicylic acid, tea tree oil, and niacinamide to control breakouts.

Luxury:

Lancer Skincare The Method: Cleanse Blemish Control

Erno Laszlo Anti-Blemish Beta Wash

La Prairie Advanced Marine Biology Foaming Mousse Cleanser

Omorovicza Thermal Cleansing Balm

Moderate:

Clinique Rinse-Off Foaming Cleanser

Clarins Gentle Foaming Cleanser with Tamarind

Kiehl's Blue Herbal Gel Cleanser

Orlane Purifying Balancing Gel

Affordable:

Neutrogena Oil-Free Acne Wash Cream Cleanser

La Roche-Posay Toleriane Dermo-Cleanser

Cetaphil Daily Facial Cleanser (Normal to Oily Skin)

L'Oréal Paris Go 360° Clean Anti-Breakout Facial Cleanser

Bioré Blemish Fighting Ice Cleanser

Lancer Ethnicity Scale Guidelines for Acne Home Care

You have to become aware of your own biology and the way your skin responds to treatment. If you have acne, your skin is already overstimulated. Your goal is to calm inflammation, not to aggravate it. Be patient. Your skin will improve.

Recommended Moisturizers for Blemished Skin

Your nourishing cream should work to maximize cellular function while reducing blemishes.

Luxury:

Lancer Skincare The Method: Nourish Blemish Control

Erno Laszlo Light Controlling Lotion

Boscia Oil-Free Daily Hydration SPF 15

Sisley Lotion with Tropical Resins for Combination/Oily Skin

La Prairie Cellular Refining Lotion

Moderate:

Clinique Moisturizing Gel

Clarins Hydra-Matte Lotion

Kiehl's Ultra Facial Oil-Free Gel-Cream

Orlane Astringent Purifying Lotion

Affordable:

Neutrogena Oil-Free Moisture with SPF 35

Cetaphil Moisturizing Cream

Garnier Nutritioniste Refreshing Gel-Cream

Introduce new products to your skin care routine gradually. See how your skin reacts. Slow down if your skin turns red or burns.

LES I or II: If you have very fair, sensitive, inflamed skin, you should begin the program by polishing your skin on alternate nights. Gradually work up to polishing in the morning and at night.

LES III or IV: If your skin is in the medium-tone range, polish nightly five out of seven nights.

LES IV or V: Olive and darker skins have a highly amped-up scarring response. Add the polish step to your regimen very slowly. Begin by exfoliating just one evening a week. There is no hurry. You do not want to irritate your skin further.

Sometimes home care can take you only so far. If acne breakouts persist after two or three months, it is essential for you to see a dermatologist. There are many treatment options that can be tailored to your condition.

When Home Care Is Not Enough: Medications to Clear Up Your Skin

If your acne persists and you see scarring and discoloration, you will need more than over-the-counter remedies to heal your skin. A dermatologist will prescribe one or more of the following medications for you:

* Topical retinoids, containing vitamin A derivatives, are the first-line therapy to treat inflammatory and non-inflammatory acne. Retinoids prevent

pimples from forming by decreasing inflammation and helping the oil move out of the hair follicle/pore channel.
- Another topical approach is to use topical anti-microbials to act on *P. acnes* bacteria. They are often used in combination with other medications.
- Lightening creams are sometimes used to bleach the hyperpigmentation that can result after inflamed acne lesions heal. These reddish purple marks will fade eventually, but you can speed the process. Make certain to use an oil-free sunscreen and avoid the sun.
- Hormone therapy in the form of oral contraceptives can clear adult acne in pre-menopausal women. Sometimes the contraceptives are used with an anti-androgen drug such as spironolactone. Acne clears up because the overactive sebaceous glands are suppressed.
- Taken orally or applied topically, antibiotics reduce bacteria and inflammation. Treatment usually begins with a high dose that is reduced as the skin improves. I am not a big fan of this approach, as overuse of antibiotics can lead to a weakened immune system, and can cause damage to the digestive system. Antibiotic resistance is another issue.

Procedures to Deal with Acne and Its Effects

If you are under the care of an experienced dermatologist, there are a number of procedures that can speed the healing process and reduce the evidence of acne on your skin.

Chemical peels: A series of light chemical peels of glycolic acid and other chemical agents can loosen blackheads, decrease pimples, and help to fade spots that remain on the skin. Usually four to six treatments are needed to improve the skin.

Microdermabrasion: This treatment removes the surface layer of the stratum corneum with a handheld device that blows crystals onto the skin. These crystals polish the stratum corneum. A vacuum device then removes the crystals and the sloughed-off skin cells. The procedure should be supervised by a dermatologist. Too aggressive a treatment could discolor acne-affected skin further. A series of treatments is necessary to restore the skin. If your skin forms exaggerated scar tissue or keloids, chemical peels and microdermabrasion could make your complexion worse.

Extraction: Removing comedones by extraction can be helpful. Dermatologists use a sterile device the size of a pen to extract whiteheads and blackheads. The procedure should only be done by a dermatologist or a trained medical professional under the close supervision of a dermatologist. Never try to do this or drain a cyst on your own by picking or squeezing, which can make your acne, scarring, and infection worse. Your injured tissue can become infected by staph, strep, and other bacteria.

Drainage and extraction: When large cysts do not respond to medication, drainage and extraction, also known as acne surgery, may be required. In the hands of a dermatologist under sterile conditions, this procedure will reduce the pain of a cyst and decrease the likelihood of scarring. Trying to do this yourself could lead to serious infections and disfiguring scars.

Light therapy: In some cases, light therapy, also known as photorejuvenation, may be an option for treating skin discolored by acne. A variety of methods involving light can improve acne. Exposing your skin to different types of light can kill *P. acnes* bacteria. One method uses a chemical that makes the oil gland and follicle sensitive to light; a bright light in the form of a laser, intense pulsed light, or an LED lamp is then applied. Blue light is the most commonly used wavelength, but a combination of blue light and red light has proven to be effective. There are many at-home devices available in a broad range of prices. In the office, intense pulsed light is used with a suction apparatus to clear plugged-up follicles before applying laser energy.

Diode lasers: This laser treatment reduces sebum production by destroying some of the sebaceous glands that exist in the dermis. This approach combines an infrared laser with skin cooling to target oil gland production. This type of treatment can help to even out skin discoloration and resurface acne scarring by removing the outer layers of the stratum corneum. Diode lasers stimulate collagen and elastin production as well.

High-intensity lasers: CO_2 lasers, for example, reduce or resurface acne scarring by removing the outermost layer of skin. Laser treatments can be painful. Topical painkillers are used during the procedure. You have to plan some downtime for laser treatments, because redness can result, which usually subsides within a week. Lasers are usually used on darker skin only when nothing else works, because the treatment can intensify hyperpigmentation.

Start with the Basics

Two sisters, ages twenty-three and twenty-nine, flew from Mexico to see me. They were beautiful despite their pitted acne scars. They reviewed the treatments they had received in Mexico over the years with me. The list consisted of just about every procedure I have ever heard of. The doctors and caregivers in Mexico had taken a simple condition—a level-one problem—and tried every procedure imaginable, amounting to more than $150,000 in expenses, and achieved zero results.

I told the sisters we could begin to heal their skin with my home skin care regimen and gentle microdermabrasion to stimulate absorption of the nourishment their skin needed to repair itself. They looked at me in disbelief. I explained that it would take time, but that they would start to see an improvement in short order. By following the regimen with special products designed for blemished skin, they would correct the underlying problem and make their skin responsive to other treatments. They left my office willing to give it a try.

Their skin did improve during the next eight weeks. We were nursing it back to health with glycolic acid, vitamin C cream, and a brightening agent. It was time to try to improve the texture of their skin. Though they had fair complexions, they came from a Hispanic bloodline. This was a classic case involving the Lancer Ethnicity Scale. I could not predict how their skin would respond to chemical peels. The heat from lasers would be even riskier. There was a good chance that they could have discoloration after the treatment.

I used a technique that has been around for a hundred years called manual needle rolling. Imagine a tractor cylinder that aerates the soil. The cylinder has spikes that penetrate the soil as it rolls, mixing air into the soil and making a new soil bed. The instrument I used is a drum with micro pins that aerate the skin like a laser without heat. The rolling drum I use penetrates the skin all the way to the dermis, improving the entire structure of the skin. This allows any products you use to reach the dermis to stimulate repair. You can buy derma rollers online. They work like fine sandpaper.

After years of trying procedure after procedure, simple skin care restored the sisters' skin. Once their skin was healthy again, I could focus on reducing the scarring and discoloration.

The Takeaway: Since acne is a complex condition with the potential for significant skin damage, you only want to put your face in the hands of an experienced dermatologist who is conservative about choosing treatment options.

ACNE SCARS AND WHAT TO
DO ABOUT THEM

Whether or not acne lesions leave scars is primarily up to your genetics. If you have any family members with severe acne, you should be certain to get early treatment the minute you experience acne symptoms, because your risk of developing severe acne may be high.

Your acne has to be under control before you tackle its lasting effects. Treatment of scars is based on where the scar is located, how big it is, and how long it has been there. Scars left behind by acne lesions are either depressed or raised and call for different treatments. With age, both types of scars become more noticeable.

Depressed Scars

Depressed scars are soft, saucer-like pits in the skin. These depressions are formed when the skin has lost its underlying support. There are three types of depression scars: rolling scars, boxcar scars, and ice pick scars. Rolling scars give the skin a wavy texture. Boxcar scars look like large pores with box-like walls. Ice pick scars are deep pits with narrow openings that look as if the skin has been punctured.

For depressed scars, acne surgery removes, raises, and fills the pit by separating the scar tissue from the underlying skin. This procedure replaces a large, deep scar with one that is smaller, flatter, and generally less noticeable. After healing, the procedure is followed by skin resurfacing. Surgery involves downtime for healing, and bandages must be changed at home. The bruising can last one or two weeks.

Ablative laser treatment can be effective for ice pick and shallow boxcar scars. Antibiotic soaks must be used after this procedure. Recuperation is usually about two weeks, after which people begin to see improvements that can continue up to eighteen months.

Fillers have become popular because they can diminish depressed acne scars immediately. Collagen; hyaluronic acid; polymethyl methacrylate (PMMA); poly-L-lactide acid (PLLA); calcium hydroxyapatite (CHA); or your own fat is injected to plump up the scars. Most fillers are temporary, lasting about three to six months. When scars are filled with your own fat, extracted by liposuction, the results can last up to three years. PMMA is a semi-permanent filler.

Chemical peels and microdermabrasion can be part of the treatment plan to resurface the skin.

Raised Scars

Raised scars come in two varieties. A keloid scar grows beyond its original border. This type of scar is extremely thick, rubbery, and large. Keloids tend to form on the chest, shoulders, upper back, and sometimes earlobes. They are more common in LES IV and V. Keloid scars often require more than one type of procedure. A hypertrophic scar does not grow beyond its border.

A series of intralesional injections can help to reduce raised scars. The injections are made one lesion at a time. Anti-inflammatory agents can often shrink the keloid and make it feel smoother. Corticosteroid injections have the same effect. Some patients have an injection every two or three weeks, others every three to six weeks. If the scar does not respond by the fourth week, scar surgery might be recommended. Most keloids have a high risk of returning if the surgery is not combined with other treatments, including pressure garments, injections of corticosteroids once a month for a few months, and radiation, which can prevent the return of raised scars.

Pulsed dye lasers (PDLs) can be effective for treating both types of raised scars. Treatment can help to reduce the itch and pain, flatten a raised scar, and diminish the color. For people with fair skin, intense pulsed light (IPL) also may be a treatment option.

Cryotherapy, a treatment that freezes scar tissue, causes the tissue to die and fall off. Combined with corticosteroid injections, cryotherapy can diminish hypertrophic scars and flatten some keloids.

So much can be done now to treat acne and to reduce scarring that with persistence, you will be able to control outbreaks and erase some of the scarring acne might leave behind. Lifestyle adjustments can make a big difference.

Next on the scale of inflammation is rosacea, a disorder that can take many forms and varies from person to person. Rosacea is often misdiagnosed as acne or dry skin because various types of its symptoms are similar to those conditions. Rosacea is a physically uncomfortable disorder that requires special attention.

8

The Lancer Anti-Aging Method for Rosacea-Prone Skin

Though it is more easily noticed on the faces of those with fair skin, rosacea does not discriminate by sex, age, skin color, or ethnicity. Twenty percent of the world's population and more than fourteen million Americans suffer from this complex disorder. From intense flushing to cystic outbreaks, from orange-peel skin on the nose to itchy red eyes, rosacea takes many forms. The disorder can be chronic or can come and go. Rosacea can flare up for weeks or months and then diminish. A patient can jump from one type of rosacea to another or have a combination of symptoms. Since no two cases are the same, treating the disorder can be challenging.

Typically, people first consult with an aesthetician or a physician who is not a dermatologist. As a consequence, the disorder is often misdiagnosed. Different forms of rosacea can be mistaken for dry skin, skin allergy, eczema, or acne. Rosacea is underdiagnosed and undertreated. If not treated appropriately from the start, it can spiral out of control. People suffering from rosacea—and I do not use the word *suffer* lightly—go through a lot in their attempts to deal with a sometimes embarrassing, usually painful problem. After trying all sorts of treatments, including holistic and homeopathic methods, they arrive at my office as a last resort in various stages of distress. Their rosacea symptoms have become their first priority. They are so focused on what the disorder does to their appearance that they give little thought to how their skin is aging. Some of the haphazard treatments they have received have not only made their condition worse but aged their skin prematurely as well.

This chapter will give you advice on alleviating flare-ups and bringing your skin back to normal. With a program designed for your particular type of rosacea, you will gradually add anti-aging products that will do more than quiet the redness and even out your skin tone. The Lancer Anti-Aging Method for Rosacea-Prone Skin will restore your skin's radiance and hydration, refine your pores, and reduce fine lines and wrinkles. Since there is more than one type of rosacea, I suggest a number of approaches in this chapter. You will have to determine which path to choose and closely observe how your skin responds to the treatments. Since your skin is so highly reactive, you must take care not to irritate it even more. Adding skin care products should be very gradual. If your skin reacts to a new product, you have a clear message to slow down. Lifestyle has a significant effect on rosacea flare-ups, as you no doubt know since you are reading this chapter. I will recommend simple changes to help you to quiet your angry skin condition.

THE FOUR FACES OF ROSACEA

Rosacea is an inherited predisposition that involves a dysfunction of the immune system and abnormal vascular/neurological reactivity. The complex regulatory interactive systems become hyperactive and set off an inflammatory cascade, a series of reactions that lead to rosacea flare-ups. When a rosacea-prone person encounters a trigger, a sudden increase in blood flow causes flushing and flares. When the skin is flushed with blood, vascular growth factor is released, which stimulates the expansion and growth of new blood vessels. If the flushing is not controlled, the flares will intensify, causing more inflammation, and the rosacea

The Color Purple

After seeing a dozen other physicians from Beijing to New York City, a big Hollywood agent with a shaved head showed up at the office at his wit's end. He had chronic, persistent blushing over his entire head and neck. His skin was radically reactive. Of Austrian descent, he has a fair complexion—light pink at its resting state. If you look at him the wrong way, his skin turns an alarming purplish red. This was definitely a liability during the meetings, negotiations, and parties that were such a big part of his professional life.

His body and skin were a stew of previous internal and external treatments. I started him on a skin care regimen for sensitive skin. At this point, the last thing he needed was for his circulation to be overstimulated. Right away, I prescribed a very low dose of isotretinoin, an oral vitamin A, for an extended period. But the first line of treatment involved looking at his diet, sleep habits, and overall lifestyle. Rosacea is a condition that is triggered by things that can be managed.

It turned out that he liked his martinis and spicy food, both of which can distend the facial blood vessels. His job was more than a little stressful, and these factors created a perfect storm of triggers for rosacea. He began to keep a log on his phone, recording each time he had a flushing reaction and his guess as to what set it off. In time, the connection between his lifestyle and rosacea flares became so clear that he took steps to manage the triggers better. He is now on a holiday from prescription drugs for his condition and relies on topical stem cell soothing serums for his skin.

The Takeaway: You can manage rosacea if you identify the lifestyle and environmental triggers that cause rosacea flares.

progresses. Since inflammation is one of the key internal factors in aging, getting rosacea under control is in itself an anti-aging action.

These are the four basic types of rosacea:

Type 1, ETR (erythematotelangiectatic): Called dry rosacea, the mildest type of rosacea involves flushing and persistent redness in the face, with or without spider veins. The dry skin can develop a grainy texture. A list of characteristics includes:

- Flushing or blushing easily
- Persistent flushing and redness in the center of the face, scalp, neck, and décolletage
- Spider veins, or visibly dilated blood vessels

- Sensitive skin
- Dry, rough, scaling skin
- Edema or swollen skin
- Stinging and burning

Type 2, PPR (papulopustular): Also known as acne rosacea, PPR involves large papules and/or pustules in the red zone in the center of the face. In more severe cases, nodules are formed. Facial swelling and inflammation of the eyes can occur as well. PPR can be mistakenly diagnosed and treated as acne. One important distinction between acne and rosacea is that whiteheads and blackheads do not usually occur with rosacea. Acne lesions appear on the neck, chest, back, and upper arms; the lesions from rosacea tend to appear most often on the face and/ or scalp. Symptoms of PPR include:

- Breakouts that come and go, usually where the skin is red
- Oily skin
- Spider capillaries
- Raised patches of dry, red skin called plaques
- High sensitivity

Type 3, phymatous or thickening skin: This rare type of rosacea develops slowly. Early treatment of the disorder can prevent disfigurement altogether. You may be familiar with rhinophyma, a swelling of the nose and growth of additional tissue that affected W. C. Fields and Jimmy Durante. This rosacea is characterized by irregular bumps and thickening skin, occurring on the nose, chin, forehead, cheeks, or ears. Phymatous rosacea is an end point for skin that has been neglected. The condition has become disfiguring at this point. This is what this type of rosacea looks like:

- Bumps
- Thickening skin, especially on the nose
- Thickening can also occur on the chin, forehead, cheeks, and ears.
- Large pores
- Oily skin

Type 4, ocular: Rosacea can affect the eyelids. In fact, half of those who have the previous three subtypes develop eye symptoms.

- Watery or bloodshot eyes
- Gritty feeling, like sand in the eyes
- Dryness of eyes
- Reddening of eyelids
- Itchiness
- Burning or stinging
- Light sensitivity
- Blurred vision
- Cysts or sties on eyelids

Hostage to Her Own Empire

One of my patients, a striking blond, hazel-eyed beauty in her mid-fifties, seems to have everything. She has magnificent homes in four countries and travels around the globe for her design business. Though her life sounds like a dream come true, something else colors her days—rosacea. When the pressure builds, her rosacea flares. Her skin breaks out in pustules and turns red. If she is courting new clients, she definitely does not want to look red-faced, as if she has had a dozen cocktails. Globetrotting might seem to be a fabulous lifestyle, but even flying on private planes takes its toll. Dehydration, jet lag, irregular and often lavish eating, disrupted sleep—all exacerbate her rosacea.

Even when she is on the road, she does the Lancer Method for Rosacea-Prone Skin twice a day. She knows her skin well enough to be able to put her own stamp on the program. During a flare-up, she uses the products for a blemished skin regimen and shifts to the sensitive skin or full anti-aging protocol when her skin is in better shape. It takes her four to six weeks to get a typical flare under control.

There are certain givens that come with her lifestyle that she is not about to change. What she has to do is build in some corrections for the triggers in her day-to-day life. For example, she could focus on relaxation techniques. She could spend some of her time meditating or doing deep breathing while she spends hours in the air. She could carve out thirty minutes a day for some gentle exercise. Getting sweaty will not help her rosacea. She has hired a trainer to devise an on-the-road workout that does not depend on her getting to a gym. She knows what foods set off her rosacea and has hired a nutritionist to help her develop a program for eating in exotic restaurants around the world. She is learning to balance the demands of her lifestyle with practices that will reduce her stress and help her to avoid rosacea triggers.

The Takeaway: Rosacea is so variable that you have to be prepared to change your skin care regimen and your lifestyle to match the current state of your skin. Flexibility is the key.

As the wide variety of rosacea symptoms suggest, each subtype requires different treatments. To complicate matters further, a single case of rosacea can combine several types. For this reason, I suggest three anti-aging treatment programs for rosacea-prone skin later in this chapter.

GENETICS LOAD THE GUN, BUT LIFESTYLE PULLS THE TRIGGER

A number of factors can trigger a rosacea flare-up. These factors do not cause rosacea, but they aggravate the condition in some people some of the time. If you want to get your rosacea flares under control, you have to be aware of what triggers a reaction for you. Understand that what may trigger a response one time may not always do so. I have a soup-pot theory about inflammation. Imagine a stockpot cooking on the back of the stove into which you keep throwing ingredients. If you keep adding chopped-up vegetables and do not lower the heat, the pot will eventually boil over. That is what happens with rosacea. A combination of triggers and life-stress can cause a flare-up. Your body finally says, *Enough!* That is why part 3, "The Lancer Anti-Aging Lifestyle," is so important: You have to adopt a lifestyle that will promote optimal skin health.

I have grouped the triggers into specific categories. One rule of thumb is that anything that raises your body temperature will dilate your blood vessels, consequently increasing blood flow and redness. Whether it is sunlight or an extreme workout, your skin can react. You have to stay cool if you have rosacea. The items on the list that follows will increase blood flow to the surface of your skin and have the potential to be irritating.

Environment
- Sun exposure with and without sunscreen
- Weather extremes: hot, cold, low humidity
- Wind
- Overheated rooms

Emotional States
- Anxiety
- Embarrassment
- Shame

- Frustration
- Physical/emotional/psychological stress
- Anger
- Sudden change in emotion, such as bursting into tears or laughter

Foods and Beverages

Diet is an important consideration for those of you with rosacea. I am listing general categories here. An expanded list appears on pages 142–43.

- Alcohol
- Diet soft drinks—artificial sweeteners can be triggers
- Hot foods or beverages
- Caffeine
- Spicy foods
- Citrus fruits and juices
- Nitrates

Activities
- Strenuous exercise
- Heavy exertion
- Hot baths and showers
- Saunas and steam rooms
- Smoking
- Skin treatments that are overstimulating
- Rubbing your skin too hard
- Not keeping your hands away from your face
- Recreational drug use

Personal Care Products
- Products that strip or overclean skin
- Masks that are excessively drying
- Products that contain peppermint, menthol, or essential oils
- Skin care products containing alcohol or witch hazel
- Heavy fragrances
- For specific ingredients, see the boxed text on page 134.

Medications

- Aspirin
- Ibuprofen
- Topical steroids
- Vasodilators
- Sildenafil citrate (treats erectile dysfunction)
- Opiate painkillers
- Nicotine

Medical Conditions

- Menopause
- Chronic cough

If you have rosacea, you have to be mindful of what in your life triggers a flare. I recommend keeping a journal in which you record the date rosacea appears,

Warning: These Ingredients Can Irritate Your Skin

A number of ingredients commonly used in grooming products have the potential to irritate your skin. You will find these ingredients in many over-the-counter products, but this does not necessarily mean that you will have a reaction to the product. We use some of these ingredients in Lancer Skincare products. So much depends on the formulation of the product, the concentration and amount of the ingredient used, the quality of bonding, and the effectiveness of the delivery system. For this reason, you should always perform a twenty-four-hour skin test. Apply a new product to the inside of your forearm to see how your skin reacts. Higher-quality products are more likely to be carefully formulated to reduce the possible irritating effects of these chemicals and compounds. The ingredients to be on the alert for are:

Acetone
Alcohol
Propylene glycol
Alpha hydroxy acids
Sodium lauryl sulfate
Benzalkonium chloride
Formaldehyde releasers
Menthol
Benzyl alcohol
Camphor
Urea
Pyrrolidone carboxylic acid
Lanolin
Fragrances

These ingredients do not affect everyone with rosacea, but they are reported as possible skin irritants that you should be aware of.

what you think might have triggered the flare-up, what you did to quiet the outbreak, and when it resolved. This record will give you insights as to what makes your skin reactive and the best way to deal with it. Since your log will give a revealing picture of how rosacea affects your skin, take it with you to share with your dermatologist, who can refer to it when planning your treatment.

THE LANCER ANTI-AGING METHOD FOR ROSACEA-PRONE SKIN

The type of rosacea you are experiencing will determine your skin care regimen. I have included three routines designed to take skin care for rosacea-prone skin all the way to a full treatment program with advanced anti-aging products.

When you are adding new products, I advise experimenting at night. That will give your skin time to react and repair while you sleep. Trying out products in the morning can be risky. You do not want to go out in the world with your face crimson in full flare-up. Your goal is to work your way up to the Lancer Advanced Anti-Aging Method.

Type 1—Redness, Flush

A.M.
Non-foaming cleanser for sensitive skin
Fragrance-free, anti-aging moisturizer for sensitive skin
Sunscreen SPF 30

P.M.
Gentle exfoliator
Non-foaming cleanser for sensitive skin
Vitamin C cream
Hydrating night cream
Skin-brightening treatment
Fragrance-free, anti-aging moisturizer for sensitive skin

Type 2—Pustules

A.M.
Cleanser for oily or acneic skin

Oil-free, anti-aging face moisturizer
Sunscreen

P.M.
Exfoliator with salicylic acid
Cleanser for oily or acneic skin
Vitamin C cream
Oil-free, anti-aging face moisturizer

Once your skin clears up, substitute sensitive skin care products and eventually use the anti-aging products while your skin remains clear of rosacea symptoms.
See chapter 7 for recommended products for blemished skin.
See chapter 6 for advanced anti-aging products.

Type 3—Skin Thickening

Thickening skin requires more than simple skin care. The disfigurement is often the result of years of neglect. Surgery is usually necessary to correct the condition in the areas where the skin is raised. For skin care, those of you with Type 3 rosacea should select a routine for dry, oily/blemished, or combination skin depending on your other symptoms.

Skin Care for Combined Rosacea Types

Rosacea is a condition in which redness and dryness combined with oily, large-pored, blemished skin is not uncommon. For that reason, a skin care routine for combination rosacea skin follows.

Sometimes rosacea can cause skin to be oily and dry at the same time. This regimen is designed to bring your skin back into balance.

A.M.
Cleanser for oily or acneic skin
Oil-free, anti-aging face moisturizer
Sunscreen

P.M.
Gentle exfoliator

Cleanser for oily or acneic skin
Vitamin C cream
Glycolic acid cream
Hydrating night cream
Retinol cream
Fragrance-free, anti-aging moisturizer for sensitive skin

See chapter 7 for recommended blemish products.
See chapter 6 for anti-aging products.
See chapter 9 for sensitive skin products.

Type 4—Ocular

The eyes can be affected by any type of rosacea. Follow the appropriate regimen for the type of flare-up you are experiencing, but leave out the eye cream, which can irritate your eyes even more. Try grape seed oil to treat your eyelids. Apply as you would an eye cream (see page 104).

Natural Active Ingredients for Treating Rosacea

When selecting products to care for your skin, you have to find therapeutic products that will improve its barrier function, keeping it hydrated and reducing inflammation. Harsh soaps can damage proteins and disrupt lipids in the stratum corneum, contributing to the dysfunction of the epidermal barrier. Moisturizing your skin is especially important for Type 1 rosacea, because doing so promotes barrier repair, reduces dryness, and alleviates stinging, burning, and irritation from topical medications.

A number of cosmeceuticals that help to reduce the symptoms of rosacea are:

Aloe vera: Anti-inflammatory
Chamomile: Anti-inflammatory
Colloidal oatmeal: A skin protectant that soothes inflamed skin and reduces trans-epidermal water loss
Purified feverfew: A member of the chrysanthemum family with anti-oxidant and anti-inflammatory properties
Grape seed extract: Anti-inflammatory
Green tea oil: Anti-oxidant
Licorice extract: Anti-inflammatory and anti-oxidant properties
Mushroom extract: Anti-inflammatory
Niacinamide: Vitamin B_3 improves barrier function.
Quercetin: Anti-inflammatory
Resveratrol: Anti-oxidant
Turmeric: Anti-inflammatory
Vitamin C: Anti-oxidant and anti-inflammatory

How to Ease into the Lancer Anti-Aging Method for Rosacea-Prone Skin

You will be building your home skin care regimen slowly, because your skin is hyper-reactive and can flare so easily. Rosacea requires that you build up to the three-step—polish, cleanse, nourish—method. Here is an example:

Week 1: With appropriate products for your rosacea type, begin by cleansing and nourishing twice a day.

Week 2: Polish every other night.

Week 3: Polish every night.

Week 4: Introduce vitamin C cream every other night.

Week 5: Now use vitamin C cream every night.

Week 6: As long as you do not have oily skin, add the hydrating night cream every night.

Regimen for Special Concerns

If you have specific targets, which will vary according to the type of rosacea you have, here is an enhanced regimen you can try before moving on to the Lancer Advanced Anti-Aging Method:

Enhanced skin-lightening regimen: Add brightening cream and glycolic acid cream. This treatment is particularly good for acne rosacea or hyperpigmentation after a flare. Use nightly in conjunction with the Lancer Method. Apply after polishing and cleansing and before the nourish step.

GRADUATING TO THE LANCER ADVANCED ANTI-AGING METHOD

Expand your regimen by adding products once a week or every other day. I have outlined a week-by-week plan for adding products to your daily regimen. With this plan, it will take you about five months to reach the full anti-aging skin care routine. If you have a flare at any point, hold back on the product you have just introduced. If the flare persists, return to the three-step program for either sensitive or acne-prone skin, depending on what type of rosacea you have. Once your skin settles down, begin adding products again. You may feel as if you are stopping and starting, but if you stay with it, you'll see great improvement in your condition.

When you are ready to move from the rosacea program to general anti-aging, add products to your regimen in the following order:

1. Eye cream
2. Polish
3. Brightener
4. Vitamin C cream.
5. Glycolic acid cream
6. Firming serum
7. Retinol cream

You do not have to follow this schedule to the letter. I have included it as an example. You can go at the pace your skin dictates. It might take you longer to reach the full anti-aging program, or you might get there sooner. There is no reason to rush. Since every case of rosacea is different, it follows that treatment has to be personalized. The program outlined here has worked well for many of my patients. You should see improvements in your skin each week.

Week 1: Add eye cream morning and night to your particular rosacea regimen, unless you have ocular rosacea.
Week 2: Add brightener every other night before nourishing.
Week 3: Use brightener every night.
Week 4: Add glycolic acid cream every other night.
Week 5: Bump up the glycolic acid cream to every night.
Week 6: Add vitamin C cream on Wednesday and Sunday.
Week 7: Begin to use the vitamin C cream every other night.
Week 8: Repeat week 7.
Week 9: Now add the vitamin C cream as part of your daily regimen.
Week 10: Use firming serum every morning.
Week 11: Add firming serum every night if you do not have Type 2 rosacea.
Week 12: Use retinol cream every other night.
Week 13: Use retinol cream every night.

Your skin might require more time to adjust to new products. You certainly do not want more irritation, redness, and peeling. If that happens, slow it down.

Rosacea Can Be More Sensory Than Visual

People who have rosacea tell me they feel off. The condition can be uncomfortable even when it is not unsightly. One patient comes to mind. He is a very successful music producer whose work dealing with artists and record company executives is beyond stressful. He is an LES V. When he is at a party or a big meeting, he flushes and begins to sweat, almost as a menopausal woman does when she has a hot flash, which is believed to be a circulation problem. Hot flashes seem to diminish in response to the same lifestyle changes that reduce rosacea. Since my patient is dark-skinned, the flushing is less noticeable than it might otherwise be, but he sweats so profusely that he has to wipe his face with a handkerchief. He does not have scaling, blemishes, or pustules, but his sweat glands respond to triggers. His pores are becoming dilated. This could lead to acne-like breakouts if not treated, because bacteria will feed on the excess sweat and oil to provoke an immune response.

Since he is an LES V, laser treatment is not a good option. Instead, we used radio frequency treatments to calm down his glands. These radio waves heat the matrix of the dermis and make it denser by triggering collagen production, which firms up sagging skin just as support clothing does to your body. When the collagen expands, the sweat glands are compressed. They become less responsive to hormone stimulation that increases stress and inflammation. This non-invasive procedure keeps his rosacea in check and reduces the number of flare-ups he has. LED light treatment also helps.

The Takeaway:
* Though the flushing and redness of rosacea may not be visible, rosacea can still be affecting your skin. Without the visual symptoms, rosacea is easy to misdiagnose.
* Rosacea has a sensory component that makes people feel off. This feeling is as disruptive as the visible symptoms.
* Rosacea can create a feeling of urgency, because the disorder is high on the scale of physical discomfort. People just want the flares to stop.
* There are many non-invasive treatments—and more being developed constantly—that can modify your skin's reactivity. You need a plan developed by a dermatologist who is familiar with the most current treatment options.

ADDITIONAL TREATMENTS TO QUIET ROSACEA FLARE-UPS

Just as skin care must be individualized with this condition, each subtype responds to different treatments. I am outlining typical approaches for each type of rosacea, so that you are prepared to discuss options on your next visit to your dermatologist.

Type 1

For Type 1 rosacea, oral antibiotics can be prescribed in very low doses to fight inflammation rather than bacteria. The antibiotic of choice is doxycycline. Topical treatments include azelaic acid, metronidazole, retinoids, sodium sulfacetamide, and sulfur. These creams are used for a few months until there is improvement. Burning, stinging, itching, and other skin irritations may occur early on. With retinoid use, redness and peeling can increase temporarily, and skin can become very sensitive to sun, wind, and cold. Laser and light therapies, typically four to eight treatments a year, can reduce redness and flushing. Two sessions can reduce spider capillaries. There might be bruising, redness, and swelling for three to four days after this procedure.

Type 2

The bumps and debris-filled lesions of Type 2 rosacea respond well to a combination therapy. Such topical antibiotics as clindamycin, erythromycin, and metronidazole can be effective. Lotions and creams containing azelaic acid, benzoyl peroxide, retinoids, sulfacetamide, and sulfur can take up to two months to produce results. The side effects of these topical treatments—burning, stinging, itching, scaliness, and possible rashes—are mild. Oral antibiotics like doxycycline, erythromycin, minocycline, and tetracycline are used to stop inflammation and reduce breakouts. Dramatic results occur much faster with oral antibiotics than topical treatment. Glycolic acid peels are sometimes used with an oral antibiotic for two to four weeks. Azithromycin and clarithromycin, more expensive antibiotics, are sometimes better for long-term use, because there are usually fewer gastrointestinal problems with these antibiotics. At some point, patients switch to topical products alone.

Type 3

When skin thickens as it does in Type 3 rosacea, laser and light therapies can be used soon after the thickening begins to work on the top layer. Light treatments of this type are necessary every four to eight weeks. Broad-spectrum light treatment can help on a program of one to five times every three weeks. Microdermabrasion can help treat acne scars and thickening by polishing off the upper layer. There can be temporary bruising, swelling, and redness as a result of this treatment. Pigment problems can arise with high LES levels. In the past, electropulsing was used to remove the thickened skin with the tissue-remodeling probe of an electrode. The top layers of excess skin were scraped off. That method seems barbaric in today's world with all the advances in dermatological care available now.

Type 4

If you develop ocular rosacea, you need to take special precautions to protect your eyes. Use artificial tears to help ease the discomfort and to keep your eyes moist. Stop wearing contacts. Clean your eyelids carefully twice a day with warm water and compresses. Metronidazole antibiotic gel can help, as can doxycycline or tetracycline pills. If the ocular rosacea is extensive and resists treatment, you should see an ophthalmologist. You do not want to risk harming your vision. This type of rosacea should clear up in three weeks if you are being treated appropriately.

The Rosacea Diet

What you eat has a direct effect on your rosacea. If you want to stop rosacea flares, you have to avoid eating high-carbohydrate and acid-producing foods. Acidic foods cause vascular dilation and flushing. Sugar, coffee, tea, alcohol, and trans fats all make your body acidic, throwing off your inner pH balance. Carbonated drinks and those containing artificial sweeteners like aspartame have been shown to trigger excessive redness in 30 percent of people with rosacea. Any stimulant like caffeine that gets your body going can also stimulate your sebaceous glands, which can be a disaster for rosacea. Chapter 11 discusses the benefits of eating an alkaline diet for skin health and how to do it. Avoiding acidity is good for your skin regardless of whether you have rosacea. For the purpose of this chapter, you will learn specific foods to avoid to reduce and diminish rosacea flare-ups so that you can focus on anti-aging. The diets do overlap. In the most general sense, your goal is to eat more vegetables and to drink more water.

Foods That Can Trigger Rosacea

The foods listed below cause inflammation in the body and are known to trigger rosacea:

* Processed food that comes in boxes, bags, jars, and cans; a natural, whole-grain diet is the way to go.
* Refined food such as white bread and rolls

RODR ROX

Jul 9, 2014

Younger : the breakthrough

HEALTH BEAUTY

33021026152816

Anythink Huron Street

** disks in Holds DiscXpress **

- Pasta
- MSG, found in most processed food
- Preservatives
- Food colorings
- Cheese; if you do eat dairy products, stick to low-fat, and slowly try soy-based.
- Sour cream
- Yogurt
- Red meat, including beef, lamb, and liver
- Shrimp
- Lobster
- Spicy foods
- Pickled foods
- Fermented foods
- Marinated foods
- Smoked foods
- Vinegar
- Artificial sweeteners
- Hot beverages
- Caffeine—found in energy drinks, colas, coffee, tea, and chocolate

Some people with rosacea have a reaction to these healthy foods:

- Tomatoes
- Spinach
- Eggplant
- Citrus fruits
- Navy and lima beans
- Peas
- Bananas
- Figs
- Raisins
- Avocados
- Red plums
- Citrus fruits

With proper care, you can manage your rosacea, especially if you keep a diary of exposure triggers. This might be a multi-pronged process that involves skin care, oral and topical medications, a variety of in-office treatments, and, most important, lifestyle changes that will combat inflammation, which is not only at the root of your rosacea but also fuels aging. The program I have just explained will help bring your skin back to normal for most of the time, as long as you manage your stress, eat well, and learn to avoid your personal triggers for rosacea flares.

The next chapter covers my program for sensitive skin, which is a matter of perception. What I mean by this is that all my patients think they have sensitive skin, but that may not be the reality of it. Since sensitive skin is highly reactive, the Lancer Anti-Aging Method for Sensitive Skin is a conservative program that starts simply and expands gradually to include a number of anti-aging products.

9

The Lancer Anti-Aging Method for Sensitive Skin

Almost all of my patients would categorize their skin as sensitive. In my observation, people with sensitive skin tend to be perceptive and aware. Their minds are always going, which has a powerful effect on their bodies. Their skin reflects their inner intensity. Sensitive skin overreacts to internal and external upsets. The sensitivity can come and go, come and stay, or be consistent from birth.

Perceiving your skin to be delicate involves a number of senses—visual, tactile, thermal—and is highly subject to self-awareness. Visually, fragile skin reacts by appearing red, flaky, chafed, sometimes waxy, and bumpy. Sensitive skin can be a desert landscape with no oil or sebum in sight or an oil field. It can feel rough to the touch. Sensitive skin hurts and burns. Wind can be painful, and so can cold. The skin's itchy, irritated, flushing, burning, stinging reactions to the environment, skin care and grooming products, food, and other lifestyle factors can be maddening to cope with. The irritation can remain beneath the skin's surface, causing such serious damage as mutation of DNA in skin cells and destruction of collagen. The damage is not evident until later when the problems reach critical mass. Subsurface irritation can show up as uneven skin tone or enlarged pores.

Age can increase your skin's sensitivity, or decrease the same. A lifetime's exposures to toxins and chemicals accumulate in your body. Your skin barrier becomes less effective when you age, allowing moisture to escape, which is why

Sensitive from Birth

One male Hollywood star has been my patient for years. His skin has been delicate since he was a baby. It started with inflamed rashes in infancy. By the time he was in first grade, he would develop hives if he bumped into doors. His pediatrician had sent him to an allergist. He had been patch-tested and treated for an array of sensitivities his whole life. His skin is so reactive, it's just about impossible to pinpoint what combination of things triggers a flare-up at any given time. His delicate skin bridges the gap between allergic responses and physical irritation.

His treatments at the office have to be done in a room with no windows and low lighting. When he is on a film set, he has to wear makeup mixed with strong sunblock in order for him to be able to work under the strong lights without a violent reaction. If he is not meticulous in protecting his skin from internal and external irritants, it becomes a tantrum of redness and flushing. That sort of reaction would not play well on a forty-by-fifty-foot screen.

Needless to say, we treat his skin in half measures. This actor has to drink his chamomile tea tepid and eat his food at room temperature. He is that sensitive. We microbuff his face, use LED lights for short periods, and oxygenate his skin. We apply a pressurized cool stream of oxygen to his face with a wand-like device, which helps to lessen redness and swelling, stimulates collagen production, and increases the skin's absorption of topical anti-oxidants. He polishes his skin only once a week. If he has been clear of reactions for a month or so, he ups his polishing to twice a week. His skin has always been delicate and requires special care at all times.

The Takeaway:
- If you have extremely sensitive skin, you know it.
- It is often difficult to discover a single trigger for a reaction.
- Even highly reactive skin can be quieted by careful adherence to a program for sensitive skin.
- You have to learn what your skin can tolerate and understand that it can change moment by moment.
- The Lancer Method for Sensitive Skin can stimulate your skin's immediate healing and slow down inflammatory damage that will age your skin.

older skin tends to be drier. Dry skin is more susceptible to allergic reactions, because the epidermal barrier is impaired and antigens can penetrate. When your skin is irritated, the overall repair process and cell turnover slow down, because energy is focused on the affected area.

ALLERGIC REACTION OR IRRITATION: THE DYNAMICS OF SENSITIVE SKIN

A medical definition does not exist for sensitive skin, which is a catchall concept that includes acne and rosacea. In the broadest terms, sensitive skin is prone to irritation and inflammation. Though there are no clear answers for what causes sensitive skin, the vascular, nervous, endocrine, and immune systems are all involved in skin reactivity. Genetics is part of it. Sensitive skin runs in families.

There is a real distinction between an allergic reaction and irritated skin. People generally have a family history for allergies or have experienced reactions since childhood. Whether using a bar of soap at a motel or shampoo at a five-star hotel, a person with allergies will see an immediate or delayed reaction in the area that the product has been used. An allergy is a localized sensitivity. The response is generated by the immune system. When an antigen—a substance the immune system reads as foreign—enters the picture, the immune system makes antibodies, including histamine, to attack the invader, creating an inflammation at the site, otherwise known as an allergic reaction. Allergic reactions can be triggered by external or internal factors, from ingredients in skin care products to foods you have eaten. Compared with reactions to external irritants, the effects of an allergic reaction to food are broader and systemic. The tongue, mouth, gums, and palms can burn and tingle. A reaction to a topical product remains localized.

Irritated skin is not necessarily evidence of an allergic reaction but can be a simple chemical response that does not involve the immune system. Irritation can be caused by an interaction between a chemical and receptors located in the skin—say, in the cell membrane—that results in a localized inflammatory response. Chronic irritation can break down collagen and impair the skin's ability to heal. Interfering with these processes ages your skin. The Lancer Anti-Aging Method for Sensitive Skin is designed to stimulate the healing process and quiet inflammation, which will not only take care of immediate problems but also help your skin to function better, avoiding flare-ups in the future.

Sometimes sensitive skin can be too dry or injured to protect its nerve endings, resulting in burning, itching, and stinging sensations. If your skin is oily, irritation stimulates nerve endings at the base of your pores to signal oil glands to produce more sebum, which can clog pores and cause further inflammation.

As you know by now, the state of your entire body affects your skin. Imbalances can lead to skin irritation. Toxins from the environment, food, and certain medications can challenge your liver, which operates like a factory that filters harmful chemicals from the bloodstream. If your liver gets overwhelmed and is unable to handle the buildup, the toxins are released back into your blood. Your skin then works as an organ of elimination. Impurities and metabolic debris along with carbon dioxide, salt, and excess minerals exit the skin. In addition, an imbalance of thyroid hormones shows up on the skin. Twenty-five percent of women have low thyroid, which can lead to dry, coarse, or itching skin and hair loss. An overactive thyroid leads to skin thinning, which makes skin more vulnerable.

Symptoms of skin sensitivity can be the result of poor digestion and elimination. If your food is not well digested, nutrients are not used efficiently, fluid absorption is diminished, and blood flow is reduced. Toxic debris congests the colon, which leads to inflammation. Chronic illnesses such as sinusitis or asthma can disrupt the immune system balance, resulting in inflammation that creates the symptoms of sensitive skin. If your body is not working well, your sensitive skin will be quick to let you know. You can see from this quick overview that the flare-ups of sensitive skin are triggered by many different physical factors or combinations of those factors.

FEELINGS ON DISPLAY

The psychological component to sensitive skin flare-ups cannot be underestimated. If you do not connect with your negative emotions and deal with them, you can trigger a skin disorder such as acne, rosacea, or a sensitive skin reaction. When emotions run high, your skin can act up like a spoiled child. Stress puts your body in a state of heightened alert. Every system shifts into fight-or-flight mode. Your hormones, particularly adrenaline, cortisol, and DHEA, ramp up. Chronic stress leads to chronic inflammation. Inflammatory neuropeptides are released, making your skin more sensitive. Stress also increases water loss through the epidermis, and dehydration only adds to your problems.

The condition of a patient's skin telegraphs their emotional state the minute I walk into the treatment room. An upbeat person has vibrant skin that glows. The skin of a person under stress looks tired and dull. People in a negative emotional state often lose the energy and motivation to adhere to their skin care regimen, and it shows. For sensitive skin, the lifestyle advice in part 3 is of the utmost importance.

DO YOU HAVE SENSITIVE SKIN?

- Do you have a history of asthma or allergies such as hay fever? If so, your chance of having sensitive skin and allergic reactions is higher.
- Do you have skin reactions to sunscreens, including bumps and itching?
- Have you had several reactions to skin care products?
- Have hair products made your scalp and skin itch?
- Have you had skin reactions to prescription medications, lotions, and gels?
- Has your skin reacted to hotel sheets and towels? Harsh detergents can affect sensitive skin.

If you have had repeated skin reactions, you have to take special care to keep your skin calm. Pinpointing what is causing the sensitivity can be difficult. Skin reactions do not necessarily happen quickly. It can take some time for the inflammation to build. If you are in a period of extreme stress, your responses can be magnified.

I suggest you keep a record of flare-ups: when they occur, what you think caused the reaction, how long your skin remains inflamed. You should look at your daily habits—what you eat, the skin care products you use, how much sleep you got the night before a reaction, how stressed out you are. Have you tried a new skin care product or hair conditioner? Changed your laundry detergent? Eaten an exotic cuisine? With patience, you should be able to observe patterns and come closer to identifying triggers. You have to become a detective to pinpoint what is irritating your skin—and that includes your emotional state—so that you can eliminate that trigger from your life and defuse the stress.

INTERPRETING THE SYMPTOMS

People have become more sensitized to the ever-increasing levels of toxins in our environment, food, and personal care products. We breathe them in, consume them in the food we eat and the water we drink and bathe in, and rub them on our skin. Combine the increasing exposure to potentially harmful chemicals in everyday life with higher stress levels, and you have created a perfect environment for skin reactions and irritation. Add an abundance of anti-aging products to that mix and it is no wonder that just about everyone feels they have sensitive skin. Product-driven sensitivities are not uncommon. Here are just a few:

Itchy and taut skin can be caused by cleansers that are too drying. If your skin is sensitive, you should avoid harsh bar soaps that can break down natural lipids. Avoid the poorer-quality ingredients sodium lauryl sulfate and ammonium laurel sulfate, which are used as sudsing agents in soap, shampoo, and toothpaste.

Burning and stinging can result from anti-aging product overload. That is why I have included a special anti-aging program for sensitive skin. You should keep your skin care routine simple and avoid using products with too many ingredients. For example, mixing retinoids with AHA can increase the potential for irritation. Look for peptides and niacin in your skin care products to reduce irritation.

Scaly red patches can indicate a problem with your skin barrier function. Moisture is escaping from your skin and producing dryness and flakiness. If you find scaly patches, consult a dermatologist. This form of irritation could indicate that you have eczema, which is its own disease.

Small red bumps that itch could indicate an allergy to an ingredient in a personal care product. The most common triggers are alcohol, fragrances, artificial dyes, and parabens.

Eye puffiness and redness can be triggered by touching or rubbing your eyes. You may be allergic to the formaldehyde and toluene found in nail polish, or the fragrances in hand lotions. You also might be responding to chemicals and fragrances in eye creams.

Blushing and flushing can indicate that you have early-stage rosacea. Read chapter 8 and be sure to consult with a dermatologist to treat this complex immune disorder.

Ingredients to Avoid If You Have Sensitive Skin

All of the ingredients that follow are commonly used in grooming and household products. Every one of them can be irritating to sensitive skin. Remember: The closer they appear to the top of the ingredients list, the more of the irritant will be in the product and the greater the concentration. The appearance of an ingredient from this list in a product you use does not necessarily mean you will react to it, but you should be aware of potential irritants:

Ammonia	Essential oils	Orange
Arnica	Ethanol eucalyptus	Papaya
Balm mint	Eugenol	Peppermint
Balsam	Fennel	Phenol
Benzalkonium chloride	Fennel oil	Sandalwood oil
Benzyl alcohol	Fir needle	Sodium lauryl sulfate
Bergamot	Fragrance	TEA-lauryl sulfate
Camphor	Geranium	Thyme
Cinnamon	Grapefruit	Wintergreen
Citrus juices and oils	Horsetail	Witch hazel
Clove	Methyl acetate	Ylang-ylang
Clover blossom	Mint	
Coriander	Oak bark	

RECOGNIZE INGREDIENT RED FLAGS

With sensitive skin, you should choose simple products that have only a few ingredients. If a product does not have a long list of ingredients, it will be easier to identify what might cause a reaction. The rule of thumb is to use products with fewer than ten ingredients. Products that are labeled "hypoallergenic" do not necessarily mean they are safe for your skin. No federal regulations exist covering manufacturers' use of that term. High-quality products may be complex!

You should avoid overly abrasive scrubs, especially those with aluminum oxide crystals, walnut shells, and pumice. Sudsy soaps with anti-bacterial and deodorizing ingredients can be irritating. Stay away from heavily perfumed products and those with a high concentration of "natural" essential oils. Both fragrance and too much essential oil can promote an allergic reaction. Alcohol in any form is drying, which is the last thing most sensitive skin needs. Acetone and witch hazel can be drying, too. Anti-aging products are loaded with acids like retinoids, AHAs and BHAs and, lactic and glycolic acids. These ingredients fight aging effectively, but for sensitive skin it is all a question of balance—too great a concentration will cause irritation.

If a skin care product contains water, preservatives are required. Many preservatives are formaldehyde-based. Be on the lookout for DMDM hydantoin and quaternium-15, both of which are known to provoke skin reactions. Even vitamin C can stir up a reaction if the concentration is too high.

It is imperative for you to use only the gentlest products on your skin and hair. You should do the same with laundry detergents and softeners. What you use to clean your clothes, sheets, and towels will make a difference. Your skin is in direct contact with the fabrics of all these items. You should use green detergents with little soap content and minimal chemicals.

Even Your Hair Can Be Sensitive

I have been treating a major-league political adviser in her forties for the past fifteen years. An LES V, she is the ultimate in sensitivity. She can use only Johnson & Johnson baby shampoo. If she uses anything else or tries to color her hair, she develops hives on her scalp and becomes itchy all over. She has to rely on oral anti-histamines to control her allergic responses.

Her sensitive skin has limited many of her choices. She can wear only 100 percent organic cotton. If a synthetic, scratchy, or chemically treated fabric touches her skin, she is down for the count. She has switched to a vegan diet. When she is caught up in the heat of an election, she builds in time for exercise, meditation, and an occasional massage to help her unwind.

Her skin care routine is reduced to a minimum. She cleanses and nourishes, skipping the polish step of the Lancer Method. Her skin cannot tolerate sunblock. Fortunately, her dark complexion gives her some protection from sun damage and wrinkles. She says she feels like a vampire, because she goes to great lengths to avoid the sun. She never goes out without covering up. She knows her sensitive skin. By trial and error, she has learned what she has to do to keep it reaction-free.

The Takeaway:
- If you are persistent, you can learn to manage your sensitive skin.
- Do not discount any possible trigger. Irritants may be hiding where you least expect them. New triggers develop...others disappear.
- Choose very gentle personal grooming products and keep them to a minimum.
- Do not forget that triggers can change depending on other circumstances. The context in which you experience something new is as important as the trigger.
- Make adjustments in your lifestyle to calm down your mind and your body.

THE LANCER METHOD FOR SENSITIVE SKIN

The Lancer Method is especially important for sensitive skin. Starting your anti-aging efforts with a procedure is one of the worst things you can do if your skin is reactive by nature. Your skin is too easily inflamed to tolerate sudden and intense stimulation. The Lancer Method will calm your skin and reduce inflammation, but you will not be able to jump right into the program. It will take you a few months to introduce anti-aging products into your skin care regimen. You have to be prepared to read your skin as you add new products. If there is any reaction at all, do not use the product every day. Return to just cleansing and nourishing for a week, and then add a single additional product once a week, and build up.

If your skin is sensitive, use products that are formulated for delicate skin. You should invest in the best sensitive skin care products you can afford. Lancer Skincare has fragrance-free products for the three-step method that have been created specifically for sensitive skin. The regimen for sensitive skin that follows will instruct you about easing into the program. Since sensitive skin is so variable and unpredictable, you will have to pay careful attention to how your skin reacts. The beauty of the Lancer Method is that it's designed to be adapted for your skin.

The Lancer Method for Sensitive Skin

You will be working one product at a time, week by week, into this schedule.

The skin needs a gentle introduction to new products. Always care for your skin with tepid water, because hot or cold can cause a reaction. When introducing new products, you have to go at your own pace.

A.M.
- Non-foaming cleanser for sensitive skin
- Glycolic acid cream (alternate with anti-aging face cream)
- Fragrance-free, anti-aging moisturizer for sensitive skin
- Sunscreen

P.M.
- Gentle exfoliator
- Non-foaming cleanser for sensitive skin
- Hydrating night cream
- Fragrance-free, anti-aging moisturizer for sensitive skin

I am recommending a schedule that works for the majority of my patients. You do not have to follow this to the letter. If your skin should react, stop using the offending product and slow down. You will not start this regimen by polishing every day, because it could provide too much stimulation for your skin. Do not be impatient. Your skin will be improving as it adjusts to the new products.

The order in which you will be introducing products is as follows:

1. Cleanser, nourisher, sunscreen
2. Polish
3. Glycolic acid cream
4. Hydrating night cream

Recommended Products for Sensitive Skin

Polish

Luxury:

Lancer Skincare The Method: Polish Sensitive Skin

Aesop Purifying Facial Exfoliant Paste

Jurlique Fruit Enzyme Exfoliator

Valmont Exfoliant Face Scrub

Moderate:

Clarins Gentle Peeling Smooth Away Cream

The Body Shop Vitamin C Cleansing Polish

REN Clean Skincare Jojoba Microbead Purifying Facial Polish

Affordable:

Aveeno Positively Radiant Skin Brightening Daily Scrub

Neutrogena Deep Clean Gentle Scrub

Jergens Skin Smoothing Gentle Exfoliating Moisturizer

Cleanse

Luxury:

Lancer Skincare The Method: Cleanse Sensitive Skin

Aesop Fabulous Face Cleanser

Jurlique Purely Bright Cleanser

Erno Laszlo Firmarine Face Bar

Moderate:

Clarins Gentle Foaming Cleanser

Clinique Comforting Cream Cleanser

Fresh Soy Face Cleanser

Boscia Purifying Cleansing Gel

Affordable:

Aveeno Ultra-Calming Foaming Cleanser

Cetaphil Gentle Skin Cleanser

Bioré 4-in-1 Detoxifying Cleanser

Nourish

Luxury:

Lancer Skincare The Method: Nourish Sensitive Skin

Aesop Mandarin Facial Hydrating Cream

Jurlique Purely Sun-Defying Moisturizer with SPF 15 Sunscreen

Moderate:

Clarins Gentle Day Cream

Korres Wild Rose 24-Hour Moisturizer and Brightening Cream

Clinique Dramatically Different Moisturizing Lotion+

Affordable:

Aveeno Ultra-Calming Daily Moisturizer Broad Spectrum SPF 15

Cetaphil Moisturizing Lotion

Neutrogena Oil-Free Moisture Sensitive Skin

Week 1: Cleanse and nourish in the morning and at night. Apply sunscreen in the morning.

Week 2: Continue with week 1 and add polish on Monday and Thursday nights.

Week 3: Continue cleansing and nourishing twice a day. Polish on Monday, Wednesday, and Friday nights.

Week 4: Cleanse and nourish twice a day, and polish nightly.

Week 5: Repeat week 4 and add glycolic acid cream in the morning on Monday and Thursday.

Week 6: Bump up the glycolic acid cream to Monday, Wednesday, and Friday mornings.

Week 7: Now use the glycolic acid cream every day in the morning, along with the polish, cleanse, nourish, and sunscreen steps.

Week 8: Add hydrating night cream on Monday and Thursday nights.

Week 9: Now try the hydrating night cream every other night—Monday, Wednesday, and Friday.

Week 10: Include the night cream every night, and you have incorporated the regimen's products.

After a few months, you might want to add more treatments to your program if you are enjoying a quiet period:

- For enhanced eye-area care: Eye cream (see page 104)
- For radiance: Vitamin C cream (see page 91)
- For brightening: Brightening cream (see pages 93–95)

If you see signs of irritation, go back to the start. Only cleanse and nourish for the next day or two. Then you have to reintroduce the products gradually, following the same schedule.

LIFE ADJUSTMENTS FOR SENSITIVE SKIN

Take care of your sensitive skin by taking steps in all areas of your life to protect it, like a hothouse flower. Here are a few tips that could make a big difference to the health of your skin:

- Do not drink or shower in unfiltered water. The chlorine and minerals in most water can irritate your skin. Use filters on the faucets of your sinks, bathtubs, and showers or a central filter on your water system.
- Do not use hot water in the shower or on your face. Hot water and steam wash away natural oils and leach moisture from your skin. Try to limit your showers to no more than ten minutes. Shower and cleanse your face with tepid water. Avoid washing with water that is very hot or too cold.

- Forget bubble baths—the chemicals that make suds break up oil on your skin and dry it out.
- Do not use scrub mitts, loofahs, or washcloths.
- Pat dry, do not rub.
- Apply moisturizer while your skin is still moist—within three minutes of showering—to lock in moisture.
- Test any new product that you use by putting a small amount behind your ear. Leave it overnight and see how your skin responds. If you have extremely sensitive skin, test the product for five days.
- Use only products made without fragrance; unscented is not good enough. The label should read "fragrance free" or "without perfume."
- Make sure your sunscreen contains zinc oxide or titanium dioxide, because they deflect the sun's rays rather than absorbing them. You are less likely to have an allergic reaction to products that contain those ingredients.
- Wear smooth, soft, natural fabrics, such as fine cotton and silk. Linen may work.
- Wear loose clothing without a lot of creases and folds.
- Throw out old cosmetics. They can spoil and become contaminated. It's better to buy in small sizes to keep the products fresh.
- Use silicone-based foundation.
- Do not use waterproof cosmetics, because you need a special cleanser to remove them.
- Use earth-toned eye shadows, which are less irritating than darker and metallic tones.
- Protect your face from cold and wind with a soft scarf. Do not forget your hands.
- Do not overheat your home.
- Keep irritated areas covered and out of the sun.
- Do not swim in a chlorinated pool while your skin is irritated.
- Do not get overheated—avoid strenuous workouts, hot yoga, and activities that make you sweat. Saunas and steam rooms are not advised for sensitive complexions.
- Do not treat irritated skin with cream remedies like lidocaine, Benadryl, and ointment antibiotics, all of which can make your skin reaction worse.
- Talk to a dermatologist before using drugstore hydrocortisone cream on an irritation. Hydrocortisone cream can damage collagen if you use it too long.

- Do not take over-the-counter oral anti-histamines to counteract a reaction without talking with a dermatologist.
- Increase consumption of omega-3 fatty acids, fish oil, walnuts, and flax-seeds. You will find more about this in chapter 11.
- Increase consumption of raw vegetables and fruits and other high-fiber foods to improve digestion.
- Take digestive enzymes and probiotics as supplements to improve digestion.
- Avoid sugar and drinking alcohol, which promote inflammation.
- Check the Environmental Working Group's Skin Deep Database at www .ewg.org/skindeep. The website rates the toxicity of eighty thousand cosmetic products and two thousand cleaning products by analyzing the ingredients.
- For a fuller listing of safe, gentle household products, check the National Institutes of Health site: www.householdproducts.nlm.nih.gov.

By now, I hope I have convinced you that skin care must be at the core of your efforts to look younger. In this part of the book, I have fine-tuned the basic anti-aging method to accommodate the most common skin problems. The purpose of these chapters is to explain the mechanics of acne, rosacea, and sensitive skin and to provide a practical, specifically tailored action plan, including skin care, supporting treatments, and lifestyle recommendations. The Lancer Method will restore your reactive skin to health and counteract inflammation's long-term destructive effect on the appearance of your skin. Containing the problem will help you to sidestep premature aging.

The next part of the book covers how to fight aging from the inside out. Your looks reflect your lifestyle. If you are sedentary, party too much, eat mindlessly, sleep badly, and get thrown by every bump in the road, all the skin care in the world will not help. "The Lancer Anti-Aging Lifestyle," part 3, gives you very practical advice on stress management, diet, exercise, and a plan for living that will keep you looking radiant and fresh.

Part Three

THE LANCER ANTI-AGING LIFESTYLE

10

Quiet Your Mind, Calm Your Body

Radiance is more than skin-deep, as I have indicated repeatedly up to this point. Now is the time to focus on slowing down the aging process internally. All the skin care in the world will not make a lasting difference if you do not maintain your emotional and physical health. If you are tired, depressed, or tense, or if you cannot sleep, your glow will fade. If you're addicted to sugar, consider fast food a treat, or cannot fit exercise into your busy life, you will look pasty and feel worse. Your health will go on a downward spiral along with your looks. The Lancer Anti-Aging Lifestyle will get you back on track.

My philosophy of self-care is grounded in the need for you to make conscious choices about the way you live your life, from your emotions and attitude to your diet and physical activity. This section of the book provides you with a practical plan for achieving total rejuvenation. You will learn to change habits that drain you and accelerate aging, replacing them with practices that restore your vitality, optimism, and joie de vivre.

Your mind and body are intimately connected. The brain is the power source, the commander, the CEO, and the control center that regulates and oversees all the functions of your body. Your brain responds to signals it receives from various messengers in your body and your emotions, then directs your whole body down to your cells to act accordingly. Your brain interprets an emotion as a message to act. Feeling anger, anxiety, fear, guilt, shame, sadness, grief, envy, jealousy, or any negative emotion can signal the brain to trigger a physical response that will put your body into overdrive. The intensity of what you think and feel dictates the degree of the response. This is where stress enters the picture.

STRESS AND THE NEVER-ENDING TO-DO LIST

So many of my patients tell me they never feel they have enough time to do all that they need to do. Most people would agree. They race from one activity to another while in the back of their minds they are thinking about what has to get done next. They are wound up and just keep going until they collapse at the end of the day. People today are juggling so many roles that they feel stretched to the limit and unable to relax.

Stress is a fundamental part of life today. It takes conscious effort to slow down. This chapter provides you with strategies and techniques for calming your revved-up brain and body. Learning to manage your stress is necessary if you want to look and feel younger and stay healthy.

Stress is at the core of accelerated aging. Unrelieved stress is associated with most illnesses. Stress has been linked to the six leading causes of death: heart disease, cancer, lung ailments, accidents, liver disease, and suicide. When stress is unrelenting, it wears down your body, mind, and spirit.

Not all stress is destructive. Traumatic events and challenging situations can cause acute stress. This sort of stress sometimes can give you an edge that enables you to deliver a dynamic speech or meet a tight deadline. When you are finished, you have a sense of accomplishment. The difference between the two types of stress is that in acute situations, the stress ends. With chronic stress, there is no letup, which depletes you.

What you think and how you react to situations cause your brain to put your body into action. The good news is that you can control your thoughts and reactions to avoid a stress response and the imbalance that follows. It is important for you to understand how your body reacts to stress and why the reaction can become toxic.

WHAT HAPPENS WHEN THE STRESS RESPONSE KICKS IN

Your brain interprets your environment. When you are psychologically stressed, your brain activates a series of responses that are meant to protect you from a physical threat. This response, called the fight-or-flight response, is hardwired into the most primitive part of your brain to provide immediate protection from bodily harm. When your brain perceives danger, your body is ready for action. The fight-or-flight response creates a state of arousal and vigilance that provides extra energy. Your heart rate increases, the systems not essential for immediate survival shut down, your breathing speeds up to increase oxygen in the blood, and your metabolism ramps up for instant energy. This response evolved to deal with short periods of physical stress.

The problem is that your body can react to emotional stress as if it's a physical threat. You are not likely to be chased by a bear in the parking lot of your local mall. Neither flight nor fight will lead you away from danger when the threat is in your own mind. You do not need large bursts of physical energy to deal with unpaid bills or problems at the office. Being on alert in fight-or-flight mode all the time wears down every system in your body. The aim of this chapter is to give you the tools to control the way you react to stressful situations to avoid activating this response.

When you react to a perceived threat, your body produces cortisol—the major stress hormone—and adrenaline (epinephrine), which turns up the power in your nervous system. With chronic stress, your body does not return to normal. Having high cortisol levels for prolonged periods can have disastrous effects. Cortisol acts to constrict blood vessels, and blood pressure rises as the body attempts to get more oxygen to the muscles. Cortisol blocks insulin from doing its job. Blood sugar levels rise to provide the body with a quick energy source. A sustained high level of cortisol results in runaway inflammation. Being chronically stressed not only ages you prematurely, but also increases your risk of developing obesity, heart disease, Alzheimer's, diabetes, depression, asthma, and gastrointestinal problems. It is not an exaggeration to say that stress kills.

STRESS AND PREMATURE AGING

Chronic stress promotes premature aging. Researchers have found that people who live with chronic stress suffer premature shortening of the telomeres, the protective caps at the ends of chromosomes that protect DNA, particularly in cells of the immune system. When DNA is involved in this way, the aging cycle can be accelerated by as much as six years.

The Skin–Mind Connection

Your skin has a vitally important role in communication, acting as the interface among the environment, body, and mind. The relationship between the skin and the central nervous system is a close one. During the development of a fetus in the womb, the brain and skin are derived from the same ectodermic cells. The skin is rich with nerves that send signals to the brain, which receives and interprets the messages. The skin is sensitive to the same signals that cause the stress response. The cells of the skin can generate the production of cortisol. As your body becomes inflamed, so does your skin. After ultraviolet rays, stress is the second greatest factor in skin aging.

Some people appear to be hardwired for their emotions to trigger skin problems. Acne, rosacea, sensitive skin, psoriasis, eczema, and hair loss are all aggravated by stress. For some people, skin is the target organ that channels stress; for others it might be the cardiovascular system. No matter what, stress will have a physical effect in some way.

What Stress Does to Your Skin

Naturally, everyone responds differently to stress, but no one escapes scot-free. Even mild stress compromises your skin's repair mechanism, which the Lancer Method is trying to stimulate. Here are some of the ways stress can show up in your complexion:

Dryness and dullness: Excess cortisol decreases hyaluronic acid, which is a natural moisturizer. Chronic stress impairs the skin's lipid barrier, leading to epidermal water loss.

Clogged pores and acne: Cortisol can stimulate oil production, and you know what excess oil can do to the skin.

Fine lines: Cortisol triggers the elevation of blood sugar, which causes glycation, one of the key actions that cause internal aging. Glycation damages collagen and elastin.

Stress wrinkles: Constant muscle tension, such as frowning or furrowing your eyebrows, can lead to wrinkling.

Dullness and sallowness: Adrenaline activated in the fight-or-flight response decreases blood flow to the skin by clamping the blood vessels, which deprives the skin of nutrients and oxygen. Such sluggish circulation results in a sallow, pale complexion and toxic buildup.

Paleness: Cortisol weakens the immune system, making some skin more vulnerable to pollutants. A weakened immune system can make the skin less protected from the effects of UV light, resulting in early skin cancer.

Redness and itchiness: When reactive blood vessels open widely, blood flow increases and the skin reddens. Stress triggers rosacea. Cortisol also triggers the production of neuropeptides from nerve endings; this can cause redness.

Flakiness and scaliness: The T cells of the immune system can over-react, causing cells to turn over too fast. This overreaction can lead to a buildup of dead cells on the surface of the skin.

Sagginess and thinness: You normally lose 1 percent of collagen every year after the age of twenty. Stress accelerates collagen loss, because a by-product of excess cortisol is inflammation, which breaks up collagen and elastin.

When you see the reactions that stress sets off in your skin, you will be relieved to know that there are many things you can do to push the off button. It all begins with recognizing how stressed you are.

THE PSYCHOLOGY OF STRESS

Your perception is what makes a situation stressful. The way you assess a problem and judge your ability to deal with it is the source of stress. The interaction between you and the outside world is colored by the way you interpret a situation. Situations that are most likely to stress you out involve success or failure, rejection or acceptance, gain or loss, well-being or distress.

The first step to controlling your stress is recognizing how your mind-set contributes to your tension. When a situation triggers any sort of anger, anxiety, fear, guilt, shame, sadness, or negative emotions that intensify stress, how do you react? Do you have a knee-jerk response? Is it warranted?

In order to reduce stress, you should aim to better control and assess your reactions, to be able to say to yourself, *There I go again*. Think about it: Is your response overly rigid? Does it help solve the problem at hand? When you can identify your response and the emotions behind it, you can learn to evaluate and to stop those knee-jerk reactions. Once you can see that your mind-set is causing you to overreact, you can prevent your body from responding. The goal is to change that automatic reaction consciously, so that you can deal with challenges with a minimum of stress.

Stress Will Kill You

When I think of stress, I am reminded of what one of my patients went through during a very intense, anxiety-provoking period of her life. Married to a producer, she was living through the launch of a big movie that went a hundred million dollars over budget. She is in her mid-fifties, an LES II. She came to the office two weeks before the film was to open. She was a wreck, emotionally and physically. She looked sallow, wrinkled, and dehydrated. Her hair looked limp, and her fingernails were brittle. She confessed that she had been inconsistent with her skin care.

The film bombed. Two weeks after the disastrous opening, she was back in the office looking ten times worse. She was gaining weight from the breast line down. It was as if all the fullness of her face and neck were being pulled down by gravity. Her face was drooping and her jawline falling into her neck.

The movie was two hundred million in the red. She was reeling from the pressure and starting to feel hopeless. Every time the film's failure was mentioned in the media, she went into a tailspin. She could not appear to be caving under the stress. She had to look unfazed for the Hollywood poker game involved in recouping the loss. She came regularly for stem cell facials, red LED light therapy, and power peeling.

The movie was re-released and the loss was reduced to twenty-five to thirty million. When the film went to pay-for-view, she started picking up. She continued with her skin care. Months later, she looked as if she had been to the skin equivalent of the Betty Ford Center.

The Takeaway: It does not take a dermatologist to detect stress on a person's skin, hair, and nails. Attitude is key to survival in all dimensions.

IS THE GLASS HALF FULL OR HALF EMPTY?

The way you interpret events is at the root of your expectations. You judge situations as good or bad, positive or negative. Most people are either optimists or pessimists. Optimists are cheerful and confident that they can rise to any challenge.

Pessimists envision the worst-case scenario. A realistic sense of optimism can be motivating, but an excess of optimism can deny reality and lead you to waste time and energy. A little pessimism is a good reality check, but extreme pessimism can be depressing and limiting. You can be an optimist at the workplace and a pessimist at home, but usually your predominant outlook will be one or the other.

Optimism makes people feel better about life, but pessimism has some advantages, too. Thinking the worst can help pessimists cope with the world. These different worldviews motivate people in different ways. Life is unpredictable. To cope, some choose optimism and are motivated to try again. For pessimists, thinking about what could go wrong is a protection for when things do go wrong.

A Wake-Up Call

One of my patients is an example of someone who seems to be doing everything right. I have been treating R.N. for only two or three years and see her no more than three times a year. Unaware of the details of her story, I was surprised to discover that what she has gone through perfectly illustrates another of my major themes. Her focus on a minor flaw led her to try cosmetic surgery ten years ago. The procedure nearly killed her. I want to share her story with you.

According to R.N., by her mid-thirties she was successful, yet still lacked confidence. She became anorexic. In Los Angeles, people saw her as enviably thin.

She decided that she needed to fix her nose, which had been broken in her teens and leaned almost imperceptibly to the right. What was touted as a routine surgery was a disaster. A piece of bone chipped off during the procedure, went undiagnosed for three months, and resulted in an abscess and antibiotic-resistant osteomyelitis near her eye. She was told that she might not live, especially if she did not make an effort to recover from anorexia at the same time she was having medical interventions to treat the staph. She underwent three surgeries, spent nine months on an IV PICC line to her heart, and suffered partial blindness for six months due to a blood clot.

Figuratively speaking, she learned to see in the darkness. She discovered the connections among her body, mind, feelings, and spirit while she recuperated. She realized she needed to change not only her behavior—for example, how she ate—but also her thinking. Over the years, her thoughts had become negative. She decided to focus on fixing her thinking. In addition to meditation and writing to develop clarity, she learned to cultivate positive and loving thoughts.

The Takeaway: Your body and your feelings are not separate. By connecting to both through meditation and learning to accept them, you will be able to navigate your life with greater clarity and strength.

A pessimist is rarely disappointed. Combining a pessimistic assessment with an optimistic attitude might be an effective way to reduce stress.

People with an optimistic worldview regard a problem as a temporary setback that is specific to one situation, and not their fault. When you view a problem as an isolated, temporary event, bad situations have less impact. You are more likely to do something about the problem. Since you do something to resolve the problem, the situation becomes temporary. Your belief in yourself and in your ability to make good things happen is affirmed. Several studies have confirmed this point. Optimistic salespeople make more money; optimistic students get better grades; optimistic athletes win more events. Many studies have found that people who respond to life's stresses with hostility, depression, anxiety, and negative thinking are significantly less healthy, with double the risk of diseases such as arthritis, asthma, headaches, ulcers, and heart disease. Excessive pessimism stresses your body internally by triggering the stress response more often for longer periods of time.

You might want to keep a journal recording the kinds of situations in which negative thoughts arise, how you felt, and what you did to deal with it. These thought patterns are deeply ingrained. You have to challenge negativity and emotional thinking with an alternative reaction. If you are locked into negativity, you will age more quickly. Understand that you have a choice about how you react. If you are thinking negatively, reframe your thoughts in an upbeat, optimistic way. You may not be able to avoid stress, but you can respond to stressful situations in a positive manner and minimize the negative effects.

STEPS YOU CAN TAKE TO REDUCE STRESS

You have to take charge of your thoughts and emotions. If you can be realistic about what you cannot change or control, you save yourself a lot of anguish. If you look for the upside in challenging situations and consider the problem as an opportunity for personal growth, you will find solutions and move on. Stress can compel you into action, and you will gain new awareness and perspective with each problem you solve. You can try to avoid or alter a stressful situation, or you can change your reaction. Here are the options:

Avoid

One way to reduce stress is to avoid stressful situations. Avoid things that upset you and people who stress you out. If being stuck in traffic drives you crazy, take an alternate route, preferably the scenic way. It beats grinding your teeth and feeling road rage mount. If you cannot avoid or eliminate stressors, you can shorten your exposure to reduce the intensity of the experience. You can get through anything if an end is in sight.

Alter

You can change the way you handle a challenge by anticipating and preventing problems. Ask for help if you feel overwhelmed. Be more assertive and do not let others control your reactions. Express your feelings rather than holding them in. Poor communication increases stress. Be open to compromise rather than digging in your heels. At the same time, you cannot expect to please everyone all the time.

Managing your time well is a great stress buster. Set your watch five or ten minutes ahead to avoid the stress of being late. Set limits and stick to them. Do not take on more than you can handle. Pare down your to-do list by prioritizing the things that need to be done right away.

Be careful not to pack your schedule too full. You will benefit immeasurably if you can slow it down and build in some quiet time for yourself. It is hard to stay calm and focused if you are running behind and pulled in different directions.

Adapt

You can modify your reactions to everyday hassles and the pressure of too much work. You can reframe problems in a positive light. Rather than being trapped in the moment, change your perspective. Will the issue you are obsessing about matter in a month, a year, or five years? A little distance will dilute a mistaken sense of urgency and significance.

Try to adjust your standards. Perfectionism sets unrealistic goals and expectations. Be aware if you are overreacting and try not to be overemotional. Keep in mind that you can change your responses to reduce stress.

Every now and then, get out of your comfort zone and be willing to take a risk. Do something that makes you fearful. Once you accomplish what you set out to do, you will question why you held yourself back so long.

Life will always throw challenges your way. When you think of it, smooth sailing gets boring. The excitement in life comes from solving problems and growing from the effort. The more success you have in dealing with upsets, the more confident you will be in navigating your life. It starts with recognizing when things are beyond your control.

THE PERSONAL CONNECTION

Using social relationships to deal with stressful situations is human nature. Just having someone to listen is enough to reduce stress. Seeking help and support will diminish the need to drive yourself so hard. Social contact and supportive relationships are essential for good health and well-being. This brings to mind another stress reliever that is good for your skin—sex in a meaningful relationship.

Aside from being one of life's great pleasures, having sex one to three times a week is a powerful way to fight overall aging and is great for your skin. Here are a number of reasons to enjoy an active sex life:

- Sex lowers your stress and your blood pressure.
- Sex improves heart health. A twenty-year-long study in Great Britain found that men who had sex two or more times a week were half as likely to have a fatal heart attack as men who had sex once a month.
- Regular sex reduces the risk of prostate cancer in men and breast cancer in women.
- Sex makes you radiant. By increasing blood circulation, sex gets more oxygen to your skin, which results in an after-sex glow.
- Sex balances hormone levels, which reduces acne and gives you clearer skin.
- Sex prevents age spots and sagging skin, because it boosts collagen production.
- Sex wards off dry skin by getting the blood and oxygen flowing.
- Sex improves the condition of your hair, because it increases the ability to metabolize nutrients efficiently.
- The same hormones triggered by sex that make your skin glow also help to strengthen your nails.
- Sex burns calories—eighty-five calories in thirty minutes.
- The oxytocin released during orgasm promotes sleep.

If you need reasons to enjoy sex, the anti-aging benefits above should persuade you to spice up your life. Sex and laughter go together and contribute to the Lancer Glow. Try it... often.

RESTORATION TIME

When you find yourself tied in knots, there are a number of techniques you can use to de-stress. Many of my patients find yoga relaxing and stimulating at the same time. Your concentration becomes focused, and your muscles relax. Thousands of books and CDs are available about yoga, and inexpensive classes are offered at gyms and studios across the country. Yoga is good for your body from head to toe. Give it a try—it will take the kinks out.

Massage helps to relieve tension. A twenty- to thirty-minute session can reduce cortisol levels and heart rate significantly. Some massage therapists use aromatherapy to enhance relaxation. Massage relieves muscle tension and stiffness, improves blood circulation and movement of lymphatic fluids, helps to relieve tension headaches, improves skin nourishment, and strengthens the immune system.

Biofeedback, which requires equipment, trains you to control physical reactions. The training measures how certain feelings and thoughts are reflected in the functions of your body, including brain waves, blood pressure, heart rate, skin temperature, and muscle tension. The goal of this technique is teaching you to control these functions. Biofeedback gives you a numerical picture of how your body works in a relaxed state in contrast with being stressed. You can check with a local hospital about available biofeedback programs in your town.

I want to give you a simple stress-reducing technique you can do on your own, namely, progressive muscle relaxation.

PROGRESSIVE MUSCLE RELAXATION

Chronic muscle tension puts the central nervous system into overdrive, which affects the pulmonary, cardiovascular, and endocrine systems. Progressive muscle relaxation is performed by tensing a set of muscles and then relaxing them. The idea behind this technique is that once you are able to identify the sensation of tension and where your body is holding it, you can relax it away. You will become a better observer as you practice this technique. You will pinpoint where tension resides in your body and release it. Your mind will relax as you relax your body.

> Warning: If you have high blood pressure, try a different relaxation technique. The contractions used in progressive muscle relaxation can raise systolic blood pressure. When you have lowered your blood pressure with other relaxation techniques, you can try this one.

The Setup

Find a quiet spot in a warm room. Muscles do not relax as well if it's cool.

Practice progressive muscle relaxation before eating, when your blood flow is not directed to digestion.

Lie on the floor to support your muscles. Once you have learned the technique you can do it sitting in a chair.

Let your arms and legs rotate out.

Place your hands on your stomach or at your sides.

Use a small pillow under your neck or knees if it's more comfortable.

Progressive muscle relaxation deals with sixteen muscle groups. You will focus first on your hands and arms, starting with your dominant hand. After working the arms, you will move to your face, neck, and down your body to your feet. You begin by contracting a specific muscle group and producing a lot of tension. Then you release the tension all at once. That letting go creates a momentum that will cause the muscles to react more deeply. Your relaxation will be deeper because of this momentum.

The Technique

Take a deep breath and hold it before you tense.

Tense the muscle group you are working with as much force as you can.

Hold the contraction for about five seconds. Focus all your attention on the contracted muscles. Be aware of the tightness and what tension feels like in those muscles.

Let go of the tension all at once.

Breathe slowly for thirty seconds. Notice how good those muscles feel.

Repeat the process with the same muscle group.

Move on to the next part of your body.

The Game Plan

This is the order in which you work various muscles:

Right hand and forearm: Make a tight fist.

Right upper arm: Press your elbow down against the floor.

Left hand and forearm.

Left upper arm.
Forehead: Raise your eyebrows as high as you can.
Upper cheeks and nose: Wrinkle your nose and squint your eyes.
Lower face: Clench your jaw and smirk.
Neck: Try to raise and lower your chin at the same time.
Chest, shoulders, upper back: Take a deep breath, hold it, and pull your
shoulder blades together.
Abdomen: Try to push your stomach out and pull it in at the same time.
Right upper leg: Contract the large muscles on the front and the ones
underneath at the same time.
Right calf: Press your heel down on the floor. Flex your foot, toes pointing to
your head.
Right foot: Point your toes, turn your foot in, and gently curl your toes.
Left upper leg.
Left calf.
Left foot.

The entire progression takes only five minutes. If you do progressive muscle relaxation twice a day, you will see results in just a few weeks' time.

Spot-Checking

During the day, you can do spot checks on your tension level.

If your neck and shoulders are tense after a day at the computer, reduce the tension by lifting your shoulders up to your ears then relaxing them. Repeat the contraction several times.

If you are grinding your teeth or furrowing your brow, you can work on your face.

Some people hold tension in their core by holding their stomach muscles rigid. Pull those muscles in even more tightly, pressing your lower back to the chair or the floor. If you are standing, tilt your pelvis forward. Then release your stomach muscles.

If your breath is shallow, press your shoulders back, expand your chest, and inhale deeply. Push the breath out.

This technique trains you to melt the tension from your body. Relaxing your muscles will stop them from sending SOS signals to your brain and will turn off your body's stress response.

Breathe Your Stress Away

Olivia Morgaine is an inspired life coach who uses meditation as a grounding force and source of insight in her own life and the lives of her clients. She has contributed a thoughtful introduction to a basic meditation technique:

There are many forms of secular and religious meditation with varying emphasis and goals. The traditions almost all share the underlying themes that meditation is an opportunity to calm the body, mind, and emotions, to focus on being fully present, and to cultivate insight. Meditation is a practice that reduces stress and improves your sense of well-being and attitude toward life. There is no need to embrace a particular religion or worldview in order to practice meditation. An approach that is simple and holistic is best. If you are stuck in traffic, the baby is crying, or you just got into an argument with your partner, do not despair. Meditation can help.

Healing breath is a great introduction to meditation that will help you to center yourself. Once you have experienced the benefits of this simple meditation, you may want to explore different techniques.

Breath

Like the tides of the ocean, the breath moves in and out, dynamic and soothing.

A great place to begin meditating, regardless of your natural tendencies, is by focusing on the breath, because the breath uniquely bridges our mental, physical, and emotional landscapes. Engaging the breath is so simple that you can do it almost anytime, anywhere. You can always find a few minutes in your day. The benefits of simple breath meditation are usually immediate.

Practice

Find someplace where you can sit or stand reasonably undisturbed for a few minutes. To begin, consciously take in a huge breath and let it out completely. Repeat a couple of times, until you feel some relief and the sensation of coming into the present moment. Now simply notice your breath. Do not manipulate it or do anything with it. Simply notice it the way you would the tides moving in and out across the beach. Feel it the way you would the tides shifting over your feet if you were standing in the ocean. Experience the length, the fullness, and the texture of your breath. If thoughts arise, simply come back to the experience of your breath, witness it, and feel it.

As your mind begins to calm, you can use your awareness, tethered to your breath like a searchlight, to scan your body for any areas of tension. Sometimes an area in your body will grab your attention, such as major tightness in your shoulders. If so, be willing to release the tension and let it flow out on the out breath. Maybe there is an area that feels stuck and dense, for example, in your belly. On the in breath, send a sensation of freedom and opening into that area.

(continued)

If you are not able to assess areas of your body that feel tense or stuck, you may begin at the crown of your head and methodically scan down to your toes—taking note of any tension in your skull, between your eyes, jaw, tongue, throat, neck, shoulders, arms and hands, chest, belly, pelvis and hips, thighs, legs, and feet. Exhale; release what you are holding on to, or what is holding on to you. Inhale, bringing in vitality and space.

This breath-centered practice simultaneously calms the mind and soothes the body. You can enjoy benefits if you practice for only a few minutes, several times a day. If you can make the time, set a timer for twenty minutes. Calming breath is a massage from the inside out.

SLEEP: THE ULTIMATE ANTI-AGING TECHNIQUE

How often do you feel that there are not enough hours in the day to accomplish what you need to get done? Do you try to extend your day by staying up later or getting up earlier? Do you lie in bed with your mind racing, unable to relax? Do you wake up in the middle of the night thinking about something that happened that day or anticipating the next? Judging from my patients, chronic sleep loss is very common these days. Though stress may keep you up, not getting enough sleep will only make handling stress more difficult.

When you are in your twenties, you can party all night and wake up looking fresh—for a while. But damage is being done that does not show yet. As you age, even a night of insufficient sleep shows on your tired skin, which sags, bags, and dulls. Insomnia can make a person look ten years older, because of stress-induced changes in facial tissue. The need for enough restorative sleep goes beyond your looks, mood, and energy level. Poor sleep can lead to increased stress hormones and inflammation. Chronic sleep problems have been linked to high blood pressure, heart disease, diabetes, and depression.

Beauty Sleep

The term *beauty sleep* is more than an expression. Of course, everyone looks better after a good night's sleep, but this observation is backed by science. Here are some reasons why not getting enough sleep ages your skin:

- Collagen production is accelerated during sleep. If you do not get enough sleep, not enough collagen is produced to replace what inflammation breaks down.
- As the body settles into the deepest stage of rest, growth hormones peak and stimulate cell and tissue repair. Without enough deep sleep, the repair process of your skin will be slowed, resulting in aging.
- Not getting enough sleep aggravates existing skin conditions. The increased inflammation leads to acne breakouts and increased skin sensitivity.
- Increased inflammation due to sleep deprivation affects the body's ability to regulate the immune system. Not only will you get sick more often, but immune-related skin diseases like psoriasis and eczema will flare up.
- During sleep, hydration rebalances. When you do not get adequate sleep, inflammation breaks down hyaluronic acid. The loss of hyaluronic acid weakens the skin barrier, allowing for trans-epidermal water loss.

You can see that sleep is a powerful force against internal and external aging. Here are some sleep tips for beautiful skin:

- Learn to sleep on your back. Sleeping on your stomach presses your face into the pillow, creating fine lines and creases when you wake up.
- Use a soft pillowcase. A high thread count is gentler for your skin.
- Use white sheets. Fabric dyes can irritate sensitive skin.

The Dynamics of Sleep

Sleep is a dynamic time when your body repairs and rebalances. During the night, your sleep follows a set pattern. You cycle back and forth between deep restorative sleep, known as deep sleep; and more alert stages and dreaming, called REM or rapid eye movement sleep. Each cycle of deep sleep and REM sleep lasts about ninety minutes and repeats four to six times during the night. The amount of time you spend in each stage of a sleep cycle changes as the night progresses. Most deep sleep occurs in the first half of the night. Later in the night your REM sleep stages go longer, alternating with light sleep.

The most damaging effects of sleep deprivation are from insufficient deep sleep. The body repairs itself and builds up energy for the next day during deep sleep. Renewing your body, deep sleep plays an important role in maintaining your health, repairing muscles and tissues, stimulating growth and development, and boosting your immune system. Quality deep sleep is essential if you want to wake up refreshed.

You learn and make memories during REM sleep, which renews your mind. During this type of sleep, your brain processes and consolidates what you have learned during the day, forms neural connections that strengthen memory, and replenishes the supply of neurotransmitters, including serotonin and dopamine, that boost your mood during the day. To get more REM sleep, try sleeping an extra thirty minutes to an hour in the morning when REM sleep stages are longer. If you are not getting enough deep sleep, your body will try to make that up first.

How to Solve Your Sleep Problems

Though sleep requirements vary from person to person, the recommended amount of restorative, high-quality sleep for adults is seven to eight hours a night; for children and teenagers, even more. There is evidence that some early birds and night owls can function fairly well on less sleep, but most people are sleep-deprived. There is a difference between the amount of sleep you can get by on and the number of hours you need to function at your best. Skipping just an hour of sleep a night can affect your ability to think and respond and can compromise your cardiovascular health, energy balance, and immune system.

If you have trouble sleeping, you are not alone. More than 30 percent of Americans suffer from chronic insomnia, while about sixty million experience problems falling asleep each year. Here are some tips to help you pave the way to better sleep:

- Set a consistent sleep and waking schedule, even on weekends.
- Start a relaxing bedtime routine, like listening to soothing music, meditating, or soaking in a warm bath. Begin at least an hour before you want to fall asleep.
- Keep exposure to bright light at a minimum for two to three hours before bedtime.
- Finish eating two to three hours before going to bed.
- If worries keep you awake at night, write down all the things that are bothering you or things that you need to do the next day. Try to address the items on the list mentally a few hours before bedtime so that you do not stay awake worrying about your to-do list.
- Avoid caffeine and alcohol close to bedtime. If you have not given up smoking, do not light up near bedtime.
- Have a cup of chamomile tea before bed. It increases the release of a neurotransmitter called GABA, which calms you.
- Make sure your bedroom is dark, quiet, and cool.

(continued)

- If noise disturbs you, use a fan, earplugs, or a white-noise machine.
- Use your bedroom only for sleep and sex.
- If you cannot fall asleep or have trouble getting back to sleep within twenty minutes after waking up, get out of bed and go to another room and do something that makes you drowsy.
- Avoid naps during the day.
- Exercise regularly but not immediately before bed.
- Avoid reading or watching TV or using a laptop in bed unless the activities make you drowsy.

- If you are having serious sleep difficulties, keep a sleep diary. Record when you go to bed, if you wake up during the night, when you wake up in the morning, the total number of hours of uninterrupted sleep, and when your energy dips during the day. This will give you an idea of your individual sleep patterns.
- Commit to getting enough sleep. You schedule enough time for work and other obligations. You have to plan your day so that you get enough sleep.

While you sleep, your body is busy doing maintenance work that keeps you in top shape, both mentally and physically. Without adequate sleep for repairs to be made, the wear and tear of internal aging processes takes over.

Once you are on a good sleep schedule, you will be surprised to see the difference in your life. You will be sharper and more productive, creative, and emotionally balanced; you'll have supercharged energy.

By now, you should have a healthy respect for how busy your body is while you sleep. The physical and mental effects of sleep are restorative, energizing, and balancing. Paying attention to the benefits of sleep seems the right way to end a chapter on defusing stress. To stay resilient, resist stress, and slow down aging, you have to build up your physical reserves as well. The next two chapters will tell you how to do so through diet and exercise.

11

The Lancer Anti-Aging Diet

I want this chapter to motivate you to take a hard look at your eating habits and to opt for the most nourishing choices possible. Just as you have personally tailored your skin care regimen to fit your needs, you will have to decide how your diet needs to change to support your anti-aging efforts. You have learned about the key internal aging processes: inflammation, glycation, protein deprivation, and hormonal imbalance. The Lancer Anti-Aging Diet gives you a way to eat that will combat internal aging. The chapter wraps up with a list of the top anti-aging foods that will combat all the internal aging processes.

Refined and processed food is the mainstay of the Western diet. If you want to slow down aging, you have to stop eating anything that comes in a package. A big part of adhering to the Lancer Anti-Aging Lifestyle is replacing dead processed foods with whole foods in their natural state. The more processing a food goes through, the more living enzymes and nutrients—and that includes vitamins, minerals, and fiber—are lost. The nutritional deficiencies that result always show up in your skin. In addition, packaged foods have low water content. "Live" foods, especially raw vegetables and fruits, contain more water and add hydration to the body. You know how essential good hydration is for healthy skin. The better the quality of your food, the healthier your skin will be.

The live nutrients that are processed out of convenience foods are replaced with synthetic vitamins and minerals. Other ingredients are added to make the food look better and last longer, including preservatives, coloring, texturizers, emulsifiers, softeners, and many other toxic substances. The manufacturers use deadly ingredients like unhealthy fats and copious amounts of salt, sugar, or sugar substitutes to preserve color and flavor. Your taste buds are affected by the overdose of salt and sugar, and over time you become addicted to high-flavor foods. The natural taste of real food does not even register once you become accustomed to the sledgehammer flavor of processed food.

Foods that have been overly processed supply only empty calories. The only nutritional value of empty-calorie foods is to provide simple carbohydrates for energy. They offer a quick energy boost in the form of sugar, but are without protein, fiber, or healthy fats. You have to learn to look at foods in terms of the total value of the calories. Here is an example. You could treat yourself to a cookie that contains white flour, saturated fat, and sugar. Empty calories are digested very quickly, leaving you hungry and craving more sugar. If you opted for a small square of 70 percent chocolate, you would get fiber, protein, antioxidants, and omega-3 fatty acids. As you read through this chapter, you will learn to discriminate and to make the right food choices to keep your skin fresh and glowing.

SAD BUT TRUE

The standard American diet (SAD) is a prescription for obesity and serious illness. If you collated the food factors that increase the risk of heart disease, stroke, cancer, and intestinal disorders, you would discover that the SAD or Western diet has all of them in abundance:

- High in animal fats
- High in unhealthy saturated and hydrogenated fats
- Low in fiber

- High in processed foods
- Low in complex carbohydrates
- Low in plant-based foods

SAD could not be a more appropriate acronym. Sixty-six percent of American adults and 42 percent of children are overweight or obese. Those staggering numbers constitute a health crisis, and the concern is becoming global. One explanation for the drastically rising obesity rates in the United States is the grossly disproportionate amount of food Americans consume on a daily basis. Americans eat an average of 3,800 calories a day when they should be eating between 2,000 and 2,500 calories per day. A consistently high daily caloric intake can result in a weight gain of roughly thirty pounds a year. But the situation is even grimmer. Here is a breakdown of the Western diet:

- 53 percent refined food
- 42 percent animal products
- 5 percent produce

This is a disaster. The most popular vegetable in the country is potatoes. Most people eat nothing green. Americans are simultaneously overfed and undernourished.

DR. LANCER'S APPROACH
TO SKIN NUTRITION

I recommend that you revamp the breakdown of the standard American diet for the sake of your skin. You have to eliminate refined food from your diet and focus on food in its natural state. The breakdown I would suggest is:

- 35 to 40 percent of daily caloric intake should be protein in the form of beans, nuts, fish, and lean meats.
- 25 percent should be complex carbohydrates, mostly vegetables with some whole grains.
- 35 percent should be healthy fats.
- Total salt intake should be 1,500 mg a day and not in excess of 2,300 mg. That means not shaking the saltshaker over the food you are about to eat. No added salt. Natural food sources have their own bioequivalent salts.

The reasons for this breakdown are explained in the pages that follow.

To live longer and look better, your overall daily caloric intake should be somewhat below the recommended 2,000 calories—say, 1,600 to 1,800 calories—unless you are an athlete. If you are like most people, you will have to reduce the amount of food you eat and avoid empty calories.

Instead of eating three square meals a day, I suggest trying four to six mini meals. Eating smaller amounts of food more frequently will help you maintain energy and optimal nutrient levels. Infrequent eating can cause your body to go into stress mode between meals. Eating small meals every two or three hours regulates the flow of insulin and prevents blood sugar and insulin spikes.

PROTEIN AND SKIN RENEWAL

As you saw from my recommended nutrient breakdowns, I am a proponent of a high-protein diet. Hair, skin, nails, muscles, bones, and organs all need a constant supply of protein for growth and repair. Every cell of the body needs protein to maintain life. The amino acids L-lysine and L-proline create collagen. As you know by now, stimulating collagen production is the key to younger-looking skin. Protein is the only food group that stimulates muscle growth. When you eat protein, it repairs the cells in your muscles and stimulates the growth of new ones.

Proteins are composed of twenty-two different amino acids. Eight of them, called essential amino acids, cannot be made by the body, which is why you have to have an external supply. Good sources for protein that correspond to anti-aging nutrition include:

- Lean meats
- Skinless, organic poultry, both chicken and turkey
- Fish such as salmon, tuna, halibut, or mackerel
- Egg whites
- Lentils, beans
- Nuts
- Whole grains such as quinoa

Soy products are a source of protein, but I advise you to limit how much soy you eat. Soy has phytoestrogens that can disrupt your hormone balance.

Protein requirements are complicated, because the amount needed changes with age. Women need roughly 46 grams of protein a day from the age of fourteen

Mercury Warning: A Great Source of Protein Corrupted

Eating fish and shellfish has always been considered good for you and a great source of protein. Fish contains omega-3 fatty acids, substances that are abundant in the brain, which is why fish was always considered "brain food." Tragically, much of our seafood is now contaminated by mercury and other heavy metals. Mercury accumulates up the food chain in fish and shellfish. Large, predatory fish at the top of the food chain live longer and contain higher levels of mercury. In humans, mercury is stored in fat tissue, the brain, and the bones. It kills good bacteria in the digestive system and makes your body less able to handle toxins. Mercury poisoning has direct effects on your skin, with symptoms such as brown spots, hyperpigmentation, burning, prickling, itching, tingling sensations, droopy eyelids, bags under the eyes, and hair loss. You want to eat fish with the lowest mercury content.

Pregnant women should avoid eating fish altogether, and it is wise for everyone to limit fish consumption to three or four times a week.

The Natural Resources Defense Council (NRDC) has rated the mercury levels in a comprehensive list of fish. Here is a selection:

Highest Mercury Levels
King mackerel
Marlin
Orange roughy
Shark
Swordfish
Tuna (ahi and bigeye)

High Mercury
Bluefish
Chilean sea bass
Grouper
Mackerel (Spanish, Gulf)
Tuna (canned, white albacore, yellowfin)

Lowest Mercury
Anchovies
Butterfish
Catfish
Clams
Crab
Crayfish
Croaker
Flounder
Haddock
Hake
Herring
Mackerel (North Atlantic, chub)
Mullet
Oysters
Perch (ocean)
Plaice
Salmon (canned, fresh)
Sardines
Scallops
Shad
Shrimp
Sole
Squid
Tilapia
Trout (freshwater)
Whitefish
Whiting

on; men 56 g after age nineteen. During pregnancy and lactation, the daily recommendation goes up to 71 g. You can calculate your protein intake based on your ideal weight; online calculators will do it for you. Most people find it easier to use calories. If you want your protein to be 40 percent of your daily calories and you are eating 2,000 calories a day, you should aim for 800 calories from protein. Plan to have protein several times throughout the day to keep your body functioning well.

DIETARY DOS AND DON'TS

I want to give you general guidelines for improving the quality of the food you eat with your skin in mind. You have to remodel your eating habits if you want to look your best. Here are some tips for nourishing your body in a way that makes you glow.

Eat Organic Produce

Conventionally raised foods often contain hormones, antibiotics, pesticides, herbicides, and fungicides. The "cides" are designed to be toxic. The hormones can disrupt the balance of your hormones. These substances have been linked to a variety of diseases and health conditions. In terms of aging, your body does not recognize these chemicals, which will result in an inflammatory response.

Eat Organically Raised Meat and Poultry

Industrially raised livestock live in deplorable conditions and are fed a cocktail of growth hormones, steroids, and antibiotics. Rather than being fed their natural diet, they are stuffed with foods to make them bulk up faster. When you eat conventionally raised animals, you get a dose of what they eat. The chemical mix can create hormone imbalances in your body that can lead to inflammation.

Make Water Your Go-To Beverage

Staying hydrated is essential for beautiful skin and good health. You need water to digest food, circulate blood, and flush out toxins, to name just a few of its functions. Men should drink about 3 liters (thirteen cups) of fluids a day, and women 2.2 liters (about nine cups). That number represents total beverage consumption including fluids found in the foods you eat. On average, food contains about 20 percent of your fluid intake. If you exercise and sweat, you need to drink more to compensate for the fluid loss. The same is true for hot, humid weather and high altitudes. Illnesses or health conditions can cause the loss of fluids as well. Women who are pregnant or breast-feeding need to increase water consumption.

Some studies have shown that people often confuse hunger with dehydration, and eat fewer empty calories if they are well hydrated. If you wait until you are thirsty to get a drink, you are well on your way to being dehydrated. Get in the habit of replacing the empty calories of colas, energy drinks, and fruit drinks with plain water. Drink filtered water if possible to avoid impurities.

I can tell by looking at patients if they are properly hydrated. The external signs of dehydration are dry, brittle skin; dark circles; and fatigue that shows in the eyes. Being well hydrated stabilizes the skin barrier, which moisturizes your skin and provides the proper medium for cell turnover and collagen production. Dark under-eye circles mean more than just being tired. Dehydration and improper nutrition cause those dark circles. If you sip water all day, you will see an improvement.

Cut Back on Dairy and Eat Only Organic Dairy Products

Most cows are fed hormones to keep them lactating year-round and increase milk production. When you drink milk or eat cheese, ice cream, and yogurt, you are getting a dose of hormones—particularly estrogen—that can cause health issues in men and women. Dairy products form mucus in your body, which contributes to inflammation. I recommend reducing dairy consumption significantly and sticking to hormone-free dairy products if you continue to eat dairy.

Cut Back on Sugar

Eating too much sugar can lead to insulin resistance (see page 191) and intensify glycation, a principal process of internal aging that breaks down collagen. Sugar can weaken the immune system. A suppressed immune system is not effective at fighting off bacteria, a leading cause of acne and other inflammatory skin conditions. Sugar contributes to an acidic internal environment that is hospitable for bacteria in the digestive tract. Consuming too much sugar can contribute to constipation, which is bad for your skin. In addition, yeast likes sugar and proliferates if you have an excess, which promotes yeast infections. The more toxins and bad bacteria that are trapped in your body, the less healthy your skin will look and the quicker it will age.

The Top Inflammatory Foods

Eliminate or significantly reduce your consumption of the foods on the following list if you want to keep your skin healthy. These foods are guaranteed to stoke inflammation, which is bad for everyone, but particularly so for those with acne, rosacea, and sensitive skin.

Feedlot-raised meat and poultry
Red meat
Dairy products

Hydrogenated and trans fats
Sugar
Salt
Synthetic sweeteners
Fried foods
Food additives
Refined grains
Citrus fruits (especially for rosacea-prone and sensitive skin)
Alcohol

Avoid Wheat Products and Other Gluten-Containing Grains

Wheat is highly acid forming and inflammatory in the body. Most wheat now is genetically modified, and serious health conditions are beginning to be linked to genetically modified wheat consumption. Gluten is a protein in wheat and other grains that are staples of the SAD. Some studies have shown that up to 40 percent of adults have some form of gluten or wheat sensitivity or intolerance. Reducing gluten in your diet is important if you have acne-prone, rosacea-prone, or sensitive skin. Without gluten reactions, metabolism for collagen synthesis will improve, a great anti-aging boost.

Don't Pass the Salt

Most of the salt in the standard American diet is from food that is processed and prepared, because salt is a flavor enhancer. Shellfish and sushi have high salt contents, as do dairy products and most condiments. Sodium is essential in small amounts to maintain the right balance of fluids, to transmit nerve impulses, and to help the contraction and relaxation of muscles. Aside from fluid retention, salt can irritate the lining of your pores, because excess is eliminated through your skin in perspiration. Iodized salt exacerbates acne. If you want to keep your skin clear, cut back on the salt.

There is no one-size-fits-all recommendation for daily sodium intake. The USDA Dietary Guidelines recommend between 2,000 and 2,300 mg a day. A lower-sodium diet of 1,500 mg a day is good for people who are over fifty or are

Anythink Commerce City
Anythinklibraries.org
3/30/2017

7185 Monaco St
Commerce City, CO 80022

**********7949

33021026152816
Younger : the breakthrough anti-agin
Date Due: 04/20/17

Tues - Thurs 11 am - 7 pm
Wed - Fri - Sat 9:30 am - 5:30 pm
Sun - Mon - CLOSED
303-287-0063
Anythink Libraries
...where anything is possible
No. Checked Out / No. Not Checked Out
1/0

Surprising Sources of Unhealthy Salt

Chips, popcorn, and pretzels are obviously loaded with salt, but salt is a hidden component or ingredient in many foods that may appear healthy. You should limit your intake of:

Sushi
Shellfish, especially crab
Condiments, including ketchup, relish, capers, and soy sauce
Cheese
Prepared vegetable juice

Prepared spaghetti sauce
Prepared salad dressings
Deli meats
Seasoned bread crumbs
Breakfast cereals
Powdered and canned soups
Bread and rolls
Industrially raised chicken (injected with salt water)
Olives
Dried figs
Artichoke hearts

---

of African American descent. The fact is that the average American gets about 3,400 mg of sodium a day, way beyond the recommended amount. Read labels for sodium content and be careful about your sodium intake. When eating out, ask that your meal be prepared salt-free. When cooking yourself, use herbs and spices to flavor your food. Note that sea salt has just as much sodium as regular salt.

Distinguish Good and Bad Fats

You need healthy fat in your diet, but the wrong fats will age you. Fat is important to brain function, dissolves and transports vital nutrients, and adds flavor. The worst fats to consume are trans fats and saturated fats. The latter are found in meat and dairy products. They raise your bad LDL cholesterol and lower your good HDL cholesterol, increasing the risk of heart disease and Type 2 diabetes. Trans fats are most commonly found in processed foods such as commercially baked goods and margarine, in which unsaturated fats have been processed to give them a longer shelf life. Trans fats increase levels of bad cholesterol, lower good cholesterol, and promote inflammation, obesity, and insulin resistance.

Good fats are monounsaturated fats and polyunsaturated fats. Monounsaturated fat is found in poultry and plant and seed foods like olive oil, avocados, and nuts. These oils regulate insulin and blood sugar levels. They raise good HDL cholesterol and lower bad LDL. Polyunsaturated fats are found mostly in plant-based foods and oils such as corn, cottonseed, sunflower, and safflower oil. These industrial vegetable oils are widely used in processed foods. They do have a good effect on cholesterol and reduce the risk of developing Type 2 diabetes. The problem is that common vegetable cooking oils contain very high omega-6 fatty acids and low omega-3 fats. An imbalanced omega-6 to omega-3 ratio promotes inflammation, which you definitely want to avoid.

Omega-3s are the superhero of polyunsaturated fats. After adipose tissue, the body part that contains the most fat is your brain. All the cells in your brain are rich in polyunsaturated omega fatty acids. Alpha-linolenic acid (ALA); eicosa-pentaenoic acid (EPA); and docosahexaenoic acid (DHA) are omega-3 fats that are derived from what you eat. A diet rich in omega-3s decreases cardiovascular diseases, lowers blood pressure, improves brain function, and fights inflammation.

Best Sources of Omega-3 Fatty Acids

There are many types of omega-3s. ALA, EPA, and DHA are important for your health. ALA is found in some vegetarian sources. Fish, fish oils, and algae are the best sources of EPA and DHA. Be mindful of the toxic levels of mercury found in fish today. You should not eat more than two or three servings a week.

ALA

- Flaxseeds and flaxseed oil
- Canola
- Soybeans and soybean oil
- Walnuts and walnut oil
- Pumpkin seeds and pumpkin seed oil

- Eggs
- Leafy vegetables
- Wild game
- Grass-fed animals

EPA and DHA

- Salmon
- Mackerel
- Halibut
- Sardines
- Herring
- Anchovies
- Oysters

Skip Fried Foods

When oil is heated to a high level, the oils and fats oxidize. Eating something that is already oxidized will contribute to the production of free radicals and oxidative stress. Oils that are reused in big restaurant fryers are especially harmful, because the fats get very thick and are hard for your body to eliminate. These fats contribute to poor circulation and a weakened metabolic process, which is a formula for skin aging. Healthy skin needs good circulation and metabolism to get oxygen to the skin for collagen and elastin production.

Stay Away from Artificial Sweeteners

Artificial sweeteners may not have any calories, but they contribute to weight problems. The body judges the number of calories in food by how it tastes. Sugar substitutes separate the taste of sweetness from calories. When you drink a diet soda, your taste buds communicate to your brain that energy is coming in, but your body does not get the fuel it expects. The body acts as if the artificial sweetener is glucose and stimulates the release of insulin. If the artificial sweetener is in baked goods, the carbohydrates and fats are more likely to be stored as fat rather than burned for energy. For a moment of simulated sweetness, your metabolism switches off, the body is put into storage mode, and hunger for sugar is stimulated. Artificial sweeteners interfere with your body's natural regulating processes and can upset your food chemistry. They have the potential to spark allergic reactions and excite inflammation and panic attacks. Artificial sweeteners are particularly bad for those with acne-prone, rosacea-prone, or sensitive skin.

Withdraw from Caffeine

Though caffeine might wake you up, it does so by stimulating the hypothalamic-pituitary-adrenal (HPA) axis. Too much coffee, cola, and chocolate can set off a full-fledged stress response and increase cortisol levels in the body. Excess cortisol accelerates the aging process, thinning the skin and creating fine lines and wrinkles. Coffee is a diuretic that dehydrates the body.

Limit Your Alcohol Intake

An alcoholic drink dehydrates your skin and depletes vital nutrients, giving you a dulled appearance. Since alcohol lowers inhibitions, drinking can melt your resolve to eat well so that you binge on salty, less healthy food. Drinking alcohol also causes facial blood vessels to dilate, which results in facial flushing. Repeated overindulgence can create permanent red, spidery veins. If you have rosacea, sensitive skin, or acne, excessive alcohol can exacerbate flare-ups. Drink moderately—no more than one or two drinks a day. A good strategy is to drink a glass of water every time you have an alcoholic beverage.

Give Up Foods Containing Yeast

That means bread and other baked goods. Candida is a form of yeast that lives in the gastrointestinal tract, mouth, and vagina. Eating more yeast stimulates the

The Joy of Juicing

A good way of upping your vegetable consumption is by buying or making fresh vegetable juice. You can find fresh juice everywhere now—from malls to street carts. Though juices should not be replacements for whole vegetables, you can drink the equivalent of a mountain of vegetables in a single glass and get the benefits of vitamins, minerals, enzymes, anti-oxidants, and phytonutrients. Fresh vegetable juice oxygenates the body and fights inflammation.

Pressed Juicery in Los Angeles is our favorite source of fresh juice at the office. Check out their selections at their website: www.pressedjuicery.com. You will be inspired to come up with juice combinations of your own. Carly Brien and her staff have been kind enough to create four fresh juices that are low in sugar to share with you.

Basic Green Juice

Toxins and stress make your body acidic, which does a lot of damage. Drinking green juices neutralizes the acid and brings your acid/alkaline balance back to the center. Green juice prevents free radical damage and premature aging as well. This juice will do your body a lot of good.

1 cucumber
1 handful kale
1 handful romaine
1 handful parsley
1 handful spinach
3 stalks celery

Roughly chop the greens and run the ingredients through a juicer.

Lemon-Lime Green Juice

This juice combines the full flavor of nutrient-rich greens with the tartness of lemon and lime.

1 cucumber
1 handful kale
1 handful romaine
1 handful parsley
1 handful spinach
3 stalks celery
¼ lemon
¼ lime

Roughly chop the greens, peel the lemon and lime, and juice.

Savory Juice

This delicious juice includes carrots and beets, which are great for your skin. The garlic contains allicin, which has skin-smoothing and anti-inflammatory benefits.

1 clove garlic
½ lemon
3 carrots
½ beet
½ cucumber
3 stalks celery

Peel the garlic and lemon and feed the ingredients into a juicer.

Juice with a Kick

This juice is high in water content, anti-oxidants, and alkalizing ingredients and will aid in flushing the system.

½ lemon
1 grapefruit
1 cucumber
2 tablespoons aloe vera juice (aids digestion and toxin elimination)

Peel the lemon and grapefruit and juice the ingredients.

yeast to cohabitate with sugars, creating a highly glycemic state and glycation. The yeast/sugar overflow causes inflammation.

Eat More Vegetables

You should replace all the processed foods with living foods that are packed with enzymes and phytonutrients. Though eating fruit is better than eating sugary snacks and desserts, fruit is sweet and should be eaten in moderation. Your consumption of vegetables can be limitless.

SIMPLE VERSUS COMPLEX CARBOHYDRATES

Carbohydrates are your body's first choice for energy. Making the distinction between simple and complex carbohydrates will help you to make the right food choices. Simple carbohydrates, such as potatoes, cookies, cakes, and crackers made with white flour, break down into sugar or glucose very quickly. A number of factors affect the speed with which food is digested. Processing foods often strips the hard-to-digest outer protective layer of grains and vegetables, the reason why refined ingredients are converted to glucose easily. Fiber in food slows its digestion.

Simple carbohydrates flood the bloodstream with glucose, which travels to the tissues in your body where the cells use it as fuel. Complex carbohydrates— vegetables, fruits, and whole grains—take longer to break down in your body, so a spike in blood sugar is avoided. Sustained energy is produced. Since complex carbs take longer to digest, you do not get hungry as fast.

Glucose enters your cells to provide energy with the help of the hormone insulin, which is produced by the pancreas. When there is a spike in glucose, insulin drives down blood sugar levels by storing the energy in fat cells. If your blood sugar levels are consistently high, your pancreas keeps pumping out insulin in an attempt to control the glucose. This stage of chronically elevated blood sugar is called pre-diabetes. If this situation persists, your cells will stop responding normally to insulin—in other words, insulin resistance develops. Among the factors that lead to insulin resistance are genetics, chronic stress, obesity, and inactivity. When your body is in a state of insulin resistance, the glucose has difficulty entering the cells. Eventually, your body is unable to make enough insulin to keep the glucose within the normal range. This is how Type 2 diabetes develops. Once you understand this, you can see the benefits of time-released energy from complex carbohydrates.

Having an excess of glucose circulating in your blood will accelerate one of the key aging processes in your body discussed in chapter 2. The sugar molecules that are not used for energy or stored as fat attack protein and lipids in the process of glycation. If you want to look younger, you have to shift the balance of the food you eat to more protein and vegetables and minimal simple carbohydrates.

My rule of thumb is not to eat anything white, and that includes:

- Sugar
- Anything made from white flour—most cookies, cakes, breads, pies, and pastries
- White rice
- Pasta made from white flour
- Dairy products
- Potatoes

All the nutrition has been stripped from white flour and white rice, because the bran is milled from the outside of the kernel. Make the shift to whole grains, which are the seeds of the plant and contain the nutrients and energy to support the plant's growth. Whole grains are high in fiber and put the production of glucose on a time delay. Experiment with brown rice, quinoa, barley, buckwheat, and bulgur as replacements for pasta made from white flour or white rice.

ANTI-GLYCATION NUTRITION

You can manage your blood sugar with your diet by paying attention to the glycemic index of food, which is the rate at which a carbohydrate enters the bloodstream. The lower the glycemic index, the more slowly sugar enters the bloodstream and the more consistently energy is delivered to your cells. Since food with a low glycemic index is slow to break down, its impact on blood sugar is less dramatic. Eating low glycemic index foods will manage insulin production. Your body will burn energy instead of storing it as fat. You will also slow down glycation, the aging process that destroys collagen.

The glycemic index measures the rate at which carbohydrates are converted to sugar and enter the bloodstream. The lower the number on the glycemic scale, the more slowly sugar enters the bloodstream and the more consistent energy delivery is. You can find thousands of listings online if you would like to check the glycemic index of a specific food. For a quick reference, here are some examples that illustrate the difference between whole grains and refined flour, sweet fruits and vegetables and those with lower sugar content, and processed snacks:

FOOD	RATING	GLYCEMIC INDEX
Bagel	High	72
Whole-grain bread	Low	50
White bread	High	71
Baguette	High	95
Cashews	Low	22
Peanuts	Low	14
Yogurt (low-fat)	Low	14
Ice cream	Medium	61
Popcorn	Medium	55
Corn chips	High	74
Pretzels	High	81
Apples	Low	38
Bananas	Low	52
Cherries	Low	22
Grapefruit	Low	25
Oranges	Low	44
Grapes	Low	46

FOOD	RATING	GLYCEMIC INDEX
Pineapple	Medium	66
Strawberries	Low	40
Watermelon	High	72
Asparagus	Low	15
Broccoli	Low	15
Carrots	Low	49
Cucumber	Low	15
Parsnips	High	97
Eggplant	Low	15
Green beans	Low	15
Green peas	Low	48
Lettuce	Low	15
Potato, baked	High	85
Potato, new	Medium	57
Spinach	Low	15
Sweet potato	Low	54
Tomato	Low	15
Yam, boiled	Low	35

To keep your complexion clear, select foods with a low glycemic index. Pay special attention if you have acne-prone skin.

FOOD AS HORMONE REPLACEMENT
THERAPY

When estrogen levels begin to fall, aging happens. The loss of estrogen has a devastating effect on the skin. Natural plant estrogens are found in foods and herbs. Eating more of these foods can be helpful during and after menopause or any time of hormonal imbalance. The list that follows is a compilation of the best food sources for estrogen. These foods provide vitamins, minerals, fiber, and essential fatty acids as well. Since I give a printed copy of the estrogenic and androgenic foods to all of my anti-aging patients, I want you, an associate patient, to have them, too:

Alfalfa	Dates	Papaya	Sesame seeds
Anise seeds	Eggplant	Parsley	Soybeans
Apples	Eggs	Peas	Soybean
Barley	Fennel	Peppers	sprouts
Carrots	Flaxseeds	Plums	Split peas
Cherries	Garlic	Pomegranates	Sunflower
Chickpeas	Lean meat	Pumpkin	seeds
Clover	Licorice	Red beans	Tomatoes
Black-eyed	Oats	Red clover	Whole wheat
peas	Olive oil	Rhubarb	Yams
Cucumbers	Olives	Sage	

There are times when you might want to inhibit estrogen so that androgens are more dominant. Testosterone gives you energy and muscle mass. It thickens skin and makes it firmer. There are medical conditions that are treated by inhibiting estrogen, including breast cancer, PMS, fibroids, and ovarian cysts. The body converts androgens to estrogen. By eating androgenic foods, you are regulating your body's natural production of estrogen. The foods on the androgenic list are:

Berries	Citrus fruits	Green beans	Pineapples
Broccoli	Corn	Melons	Squash
Buckwheat	Figs	Onions	
Cabbage	Grapes	Peas	

TOP FOODS TO BE YOUNGER

You have learned how to evaluate the anti-aging attributes of food in a number of different ways in this chapter. I want to wrap it up by giving you a list of the most powerful anti-aging foods. You should post it on your refrigerator and carry a copy with you to refer to when you are at the market or a restaurant. Incorporating these foods into your diet will brighten up your skin, supercharge your energy, lighten your spirits, and get your body working like a well-maintained machine.

Avocados: A rich source of monounsaturated fatty acids and biotin for healthy skin.

Berries: Loaded with anti-oxidants that neutralize free radicals, they contribute to collagen production. The darker the berry, the higher the content of vitamins C and E.

Brazil nuts: High in selenium, a mineral that repairs cell damage and slows down the skin's aging process.

Carrots: A great source of vitamin A, which is important for skin health. Beta-carotene and lycopene protect your skin from the sun and repair skin cells. Carrots are high glycemic, so do not go overboard with them.

Celery: Celery has a high water content that is good for your skin.

Chickpeas (garbanzo beans): These little beans are an anti-aging powerhouse. High in protein and fiber, they contain quercetin, which has anti-inflammatory properties. The manganese and copper support cell metabolism.

Cod: Aside from omega-3s, this fish contains selenium, which is a safeguard against sun damage.

Cruciferous vegetables—bok choy, broccoli, brussels sprouts, cabbage, cauliflower, kale: Protect against cancer and reduce oxidative stress. All are high in anti-oxidants and have some omega-3s.

Cucumbers: The high water content is great for your skin, and the silica in the peel boosts collagen production. Try to find cucumbers that have not been waxed.

Dark chocolate: The resveratrol and flavinols promote circulation and protect against moderate sun damage.

Eggs: A great source of protein, eggs are rich in iron and biotin, which keep your hair and skin full and healthy. Try eating just the whites to avoid cholesterol problems.

Guava: Packed with vitamin C, the anti-oxidant that boosts collagen production.

Kelp: This sea plant has high levels of vitamins C and E, which protect fats in the skin's moisture barrier from free radical damage.

Kiwi: Ounce for ounce, kiwi is the most nutrition-dense fruit. Fiber, phytonutrients, folic acid, vitamin C, vitamin E, calcium, copper, iron, magnesium, potassium, and zinc make this small fruit a super food.

Lean beef: A good source of protein and iron—but eat in moderation.

Mango: This vitamin-C-rich fruit helps to alkalize the body, improves digestion, normalizes insulin levels, and boosts the immune system. High levels of vitamin E are good for skin health.

Melons: High in water content, but also high glycemic, melons should be eaten sparingly.

Pomegranate seeds: Rich in ellagic acid and punicalagin, which fight free radical damage.

Romaine lettuce: High in vitamin A, which revitalizes the skin by boosting cell turnover.

Sardines: High in omega-3 fatty acids, promoting hair growth and shine.

Spinach: High in folate (vitamin B_9), which aids in the production and maintenance of new cells; in vitamin C, which the body needs to produce sebum to keep skin looking young; and in lutein, for eye health.

Sunflower seeds: Contain lignin phytoestrogens that prevent the breakdown of collagen and strengthen the skin's lipid barrier.

Sweet potato: Beta-carotene makes this vegetable a powerful anti-oxidant and a source of vitamin A.

Tomatoes: Along with anti-oxidants, tomatoes contain lycopene, which protects from UV damage. Eat in moderation, because tomatoes are acidic.

Walnuts: High in omega-3 fatty acids. Their anti-inflammatory power can relieve skin diseases such as eczema.

Whole grains: High in fiber, whole grains keep blood sugar levels stable and reduce glycation.

Wild salmon: An important anti-aging food, filled with omega-3 fatty acids that improve brain function and reduce inflammation.

Zinc, copper, selenium: These minerals are essential for collagen production. Zinc strengthens the immune system. They can be found in chicken, lean beef, walnuts, and chickpeas.

I have intentionally not given you a set diet, because these seldom carry over into your life once you have finished the two weeks or thirty days of extreme deprivation. You may follow rigid meal plans for two weeks and feel great. Once you are left to your own devices, though, you will gradually revert to those unhealthy eating habits. My goal is to give you the information you need to create an anti-aging eating strategy that works for you.

If you have to, keep track—on your phone, on your laptop, or in a notebook—of the calories and protein content of the food you consume. Online trackers will analyze the food you eat nutritionally, which makes it easy. Check to see if you are eating protein, complex carbohydrates, and healthy fats in the right proportions.

To close the chapter, I have to say that no one is perfect. You can have that piece of birthday cake, slice of pizza, or cheeseburger now and then. Feeling deprived is not good for you. Just make certain you do not stray every day. Recently, I had an experience that taught me a lesson. My wife and I were at LAX about to catch a plane. There happens to be a fantastic Mexican food place at the terminal that I could not resist. I splurged on a tostada that was delicious going down—but I woke up the next morning with puffy eyes and a bloated stomach. A few minutes of enjoyment was not worth the consequences. My physical reaction made it clear that I had done a good job cleaning up my act in the food department. My body was so used to healthy, pure food that the hit of simple carbohydrates and unhealthy fat was a shock. The message was clear: My body works better when I eat well. It would be unrealistic to think that I will not be tempted again, but for now, I know what is good for me.

The final phase of the Lancer Anti-Aging Lifestyle triad is exercise to rev up your circulation, prevent muscle loss, and stimulate cell renewal. I am not asking you to become a workout fanatic. If you incorporate a moderate physical activity into your life most days of the week, you will see and feel big differences in no time at all. The next chapter will motivate you to get moving and beat aging at its own game.

12

Moving to Younger

Increasing your physical activity is one of the most important things you can do to age well and stay healthy, yet the United States remains predominantly a sedentary society. The Centers for Disease Control reports that more than 60 percent of Americans are not physically active on a regular basis, with only 15 percent of the population reporting vigorous activity—intense enough to make the heart beat fast and to breathe hard—for twenty minutes or more three times a week. This lack of physical activity is creating a health crisis in the U.S. as well as across the globe that is aging us inside and out.

Some scientists suggest that inactivity should be considered a diseased state. Consider that walking ten thousand steps a day reduces the risk of:

- Heart attacks by 90 percent (American Heart Association)
- Cancer by 30 to 70 percent (American Cancer Association)
- Type 2 diabetes by 50 percent (American Diabetes Association)
- Strokes by 70 percent (American Heart Association)

The anti-aging effects of exercise go way beyond improved muscle tone, cardiovascular health, and weight loss. Every cell in the body benefits when you get moving, and I mean that literally. A recent study compared the telomeres of young and middle-aged sedentary men and women and serious runners in their twenties and middle age. On the surface, there was a striking difference in the appearance of the middle-aged, serious athletes and the sedentary group of the same age. The highly active people looked much younger than their inactive peers. Going deeper, when the researchers measured the telomeres of the middle-aged subjects, they found the telomeres of the sedentary older group were on average 40 percent shorter than in the sedentary young group. The older runners had strikingly young telomeres, only 10 percent shorter than the young runners. In fact, the telomere loss in the aging runners was reduced by approximately 75 percent!

If those numbers are not convincing enough for you to lace up your gym shoes or roll out your yoga mat, a look at the psychological and anti-aging effects should persuade you that exercise has to be part of your life if you want to feel and look younger. Just half an hour of moderate physical activity most days of the week will have a significant effect on your mind and body.

EXERCISE AS A STRESS RELIEVER

When emotions chronically trigger the stress response, metabolic problems develop, resulting in central obesity, hypertension, and high cholesterol and triglycerides, as well as dysfunction in the cell walls. Cortisol and other by-products of the stress response continue to circulate in the body as if the volume is turned up full blast. Exercise uses the energy produced by the fight-or-flight response, bringing the body back into balance. Exercise turns off the stress response by sending a message to the brain that you are using cortisol for its original purpose. Here are some additional mental benefits of exercise:

- Exercise is an outlet for negative energy such as hostility or anger. You will release negative emotions in a healthy way if you exert yourself physically.
- Exercise can help you achieve longer, more restful sleep. Moderate exercise at least three hours before bedtime can help you to relax and sleep better.
- Exercise relaxes muscles that tense with stress. Tight muscles can lose tone, but working your muscles releases stored energy; the muscles return to a normal resting state. This applies to your face as well as your legs, core, and arms. Your facial expressions may not set as wrinkles if your face muscles relax regularly.

- Moving will improve your mood. Exercise activates serotonin and norepinephrine and synchronizes brain chemicals that affect mood. Exercise stimulates endorphins, the source of "runner's high."
- Testosterone and HGH get a boost when you exercise. This fuels sex drive and builds muscle tissue, which you know is good for you.

The right degree of exercise is a surefire stress reliever, and defusing stress is essential to fight aging.

EXERCISE AND YOUR SKIN

Exercise is a must if you want to be radiant. Physical activity increases circulation and delivers more nutrients and oxygen to the skin, which greatly improves skin health. Cell renewal speeds up, and the natural production of collagen increases. Aside from keeping your skin vital, the increased blood flow carries away waste products—including free radicals from working cells—and flushes cellular debris from your systems. The increased blood flow also revs up your immune system by producing more white blood cells, neutrophils, and natural killer cells to fight bacteria. By reducing the levels of stress hormones in your body, exercise controls inflammation and counters the destruction of free radicals at the same time.

If you exercise hard enough to sweat, you have eliminated sodium and impurities from your body, which can clog pores. When muscles contract during exercise, they squeeze the lymph nodes, helping them to pump waste out of your system. Better lymph drainage moves the metabolic trash that pollutes your body.

From the time you are born until you reach your thirties, your muscles grow stronger and larger. At some point in your thirties, the building reverses, and you begin to lose muscle mass. This breakdown of muscle tissue accelerates around the age of sixty. People who are inactive lose as much as 3 to 5 percent of their muscle mass each decade after thirty. The reduction of muscle mass advances the aging process and causes a range of other medical complications.

Muscle is the body's most metabolically active tissue. When muscle mass diminishes, metabolism slows down. The loss of muscle mass means a reduction of your strength, endurance, and aerobic capacity. When these things happen, you tire more easily. Exercise will bring the metabolic forces of tearing down and building up into balance to prevent muscle loss.

Toning your muscles not only keeps your metabolism high, but also makes your skin look firmer. The more toned the muscles are beneath your skin, the better support your skin will have. It will look and feel healthier. When you lose muscle mass, your skin gets saggy and wrinkled.

Since moderate physical activity eases stress and reduces cortisol levels, the sebaceous glands are no longer overstimulated and producing excess oil. This is good news for those of you with acne.

JUST THE RIGHT AMOUNT OF EXERCISE

After touting how much exercise can do for you, I have to warn you that exercise has the potential to do damage to your skin. For one thing, if you get your exercise outdoors, you increase your exposure to wrinkle-inducing UV rays. I would never advise you to give up an active life you love, but if you are an outdoor exerciser, you have to double or even triple up on sun protection. Always wear a hat and workout clothes with SPF built in.

Working out intensely is stressful to your body. Strenuous exercise triggers the same hormonal cascade as stress does, leading to inflammation. Your body produces more free radicals when your exert yourself, which ages your skin.

It might go against common wisdom when I say that you do not have to push yourself hard to get the benefits of exercise. I hit the treadmill or elliptical trainer every day, pacing myself at a very moderate 3.5 miles per hour. When I reach 1.81 miles, I stop. I advocate a measured approach to physical activity. Stretching, yoga, Pilates, brisk walking, and reasonable weight resistance training are all good for the skin, because they increase circulation but do not push metabolism to an extreme that produces oxidative stress. Moderate exercise will help to reduce stress and inflammation.

A WORD OF CAUTION

If you are wearing makeup, you should remove it before working out. You do not want the makeup to mix with sweat and oil and clog your pores. If you have rosacea-prone skin, be careful about raising your body temperature too high. Aerobic activity that increases circulation may not be right for you. The dilated blood vessels will lead to flushing and flare-ups. It's a good idea to exercise in a cool environment. Swimming might be a good choice for you. Chlorine is very drying, so make sure to nourish your skin afterward. If you have problem areas, use cool compresses after you exercise.

If you have eczema or psoriasis, it is not uncommon to experience a flare-up after strenuous activity. The salt from perspiration can irritate your skin. You might want to moisturize before working out to protect your skin from the sweat. Make sure to apply moisturizer wherever your skin has creases—on the arms, legs, and groin—because the sweat can collect in those creases.

Of course, if you get your exercise outside, you need to apply sunscreen liberally. Sweating increases your chances of burning. It takes about 40 percent less UV rays to burn if you are perspiring. You might want to use oil-free sunscreen to keep your eyes from burning if sweat runs into them.

When working out you have to be careful about acne mechanica, a condition that results from chafing skin. It's a good idea to use moisture-wicking workout clothes where the fabric is likely to rub against your skin.

Always shower after you exercise to eliminate the mix of oil and sweat that can clog your pores.

GET MOVING

It is easy to overestimate how much exercise you are getting and to underestimate how many calories you consume. There are always countless reasons not to exercise, starting with not having enough time. You might tell yourself you are too old, too tired, or too out of shape. You might not want to spend the money on a gym or be too embarrassed to go to one. You could defeat yourself before you even begin by presuming you will not stick to it. Instead, think about how much more you will be able to get done—and how much better your relationships with family and friends will be if you are upbeat and energized.

The good news is that the greatest gains in health occur when you go from a totally inactive lifestyle to a moderately active one. Only thirty to fifty minutes of moderate exercise three or four days a week is what you have to build into your schedule to improve your health and control your weight. You do not have to do all your exercise at once. If you are pressed for time, you can do ten-minute increments during the day.

The hardest part of adding physical activity to your life is to begin. It does not take long to form a habit. If you commit to moving twenty minutes to half an hour four or five days a week, you will see and feel improvements in a matter of weeks. It takes about eight weeks for your mind and body to make the connection between moving and feeling good. Once that connection is made, you will associate exercise with pleasure, and movement will become a necessary part of your life. Think of it this way: Exercising twenty to thirty minutes is less than 3 percent of your waking day, and you will feel better for the other 97 percent. That is a great return on investment.

Regular exercise is not limited to running, calisthenics, or weight training. You have to choose exercise that you enjoy doing, so you are motivated to keep it up. For your anti-aging goals, you do not have to overdo it. You can take a walk or ride a bike for half an hour a day. You could take a yoga class with friends, play basketball or tennis, garden, or ride horses. You could have a free weight routine to do while you are watching television in the evening. Your body is meant to move, and you will feel—and look—so much better if you do.

I recommend scheduling a set time for exercise. If you try to be flexible, you might end up putting off your workout or even skipping it. Many of my patients choose to work out with a trainer, which can be pricey, but they know they will not flake out on an appointment for which they are paying. All of us have our own form of motivation. There is no reason you cannot make an appointment with yourself and keep it. Make your exercise time a priority. Whether you get up half an hour earlier to start the day out right, work out immediately after the kids go off to school, take a break at lunchtime, or exercise right after work to make a clean break from the office, you can find the time to do something good for yourself.

If your aim is to burn fat, workouts that are long, slow, and cover distances are the most effective. If time is an issue, the more intensely you work out, the less time you will have to spend exercising. For example, shoveling snow for fifteen minutes is equivalent to walking for two miles in thirty minutes. Here are some examples of moderate and vigorous exercise based on exertion:

Moderate exercise: Pushing a stroller a mile and a half in thirty minutes; walking briskly at 3 to 4 mph; canoeing, kayaking, rowing; swimming laps; cycling under 10 mph; dancing fast and hard; golfing while carrying clubs; raking leaves; skiing; calisthenics; aerobics class; hatha yoga; Pilates; aerobic dancing; working with light weights; power walking.

Vigorous exercise: Mountain climbing; chopping wood; Spinning; jogging at 6 mph; surfing; jumping rope; playing singles tennis, racquetball, or squash; backpacking; ice-skating or in-line skating; cross-country skiing; boxing; cycling more than 10 mph; snowshoeing; kickboxing; soccer; lacrosse; field hockey; basketball; walking briskly uphill while carrying something.

You do not have to do the same thing every time you exercise. Change it up if you get bored.

Ease into your program. You might need to start with five minutes once or twice a day depending on your level of fitness. You might start by walking ten minutes a day three times a week. You can add a couple of minutes a week until you work your way up to thirty or forty minutes. As you become more fit, you will want to challenge your body, but overdoing it at the beginning of your commitment can undermine your efforts. There is no reason to push too hard. You have the rest of your life to improve.

You are exercising to increase blood flow to all of your organs, which will help to stimulate your metabolism and aid the lymphatic drainage of toxins. You are aiming to maintain muscle mass and bone density and reduce your BMI. Stretching, Pilates, cardio exercise that gets your heart rate up, and weight resistance exercise will help you to achieve these goals. I have asked two of my prominent patients to create simple workouts that you can do anywhere. You will not need special equipment to do these routines. You just need the will.

BASIC PILATES WORKOUT

Debi Monahan started her career as an actress on the Broadway stage, and went on to work in movies and television. She is now a leading Pilates trainer who transforms the bodies of many of today's most outstanding models and celebrities. Whenever she comes to the office, my staff always want to know how she got into such great shape. Her energy and enthusiasm are contagious. She has been good enough to contribute some basic Pilates mat exercises to help you work on muscle definition, strength, and flexibility. What follows is Debi's introduction to Pilates:

Pilates is a body conditioning method developed by Joseph H. Pilates, a unique system of strengthening and stretching exercises designed to lengthen and tone the body. Integrating precise muscle control, one of the foundational principles of Pilates, is designed to help you achieve a body that looks good, feels good, and will support you for life. Pilates not only enhances your physical strength, flexibility, coordination, agility, and endurance but also reduces stress, combats fatigue, and improves mental focus and circulation. Doing just a few Pilates mat exercises a day will rejuvenate you both physically and mentally. Mr. Pilates believed in working smarter, not longer, a goal that should fit well in your busy life.

These basic Pilates core exercises can be done anywhere, at home or at the office. The exercises must be performed with extreme control to avoid injury and produce positive results. Remember: It is the quality of the movement that will produce the best results. If you are experiencing an uncomfortable strain on an area of your body, stop. Make sure you are working from the proper muscles and try again. If discomfort continues, move on to another exercise. Keep in mind that your strength and control will increase with time and practice. Some exercises may not be suited to your body. Use your best judgment, and most of all listen to your body. I recommend consulting with your doctor before engaging in any fitness program.

A few principles before you begin:

Breathe

In Pilates, we use a breathing technique known as lateral breathing. We expand the ribs sideways with each breath, by maintaining a constant inward pull of the deep abdominal muscles. Maintaining that abdominal contraction is important for successful performance and the protection of your body. The Lancer Method is designed to stir up the circulatory system and oxygenate the blood.

Precision

Precision is key. The greater the precision, the greater the benefit will be. Begin slowly. Stay focused and in constant control of your body.

The Powerhouse (or Core)

Your core is a large group of muscles—your abdominals, lower back, hips, and buttocks—that make up your center, which in Pilates is known as the powerhouse. All energy for the movements of Pilates initiates from the powerhouse. Imagine stretching your upper body away from your hips as if you were being cinched into a corset. This action of pulling up and in simultaneously will automatically engage your powerhouse muscles and help to protect your lower back.

Remember:

It is the quality of the movement that will produce the best results. Perform the exercise slowly, with great control and fluidity. Engage the proper muscles and breathe. If it hurts your neck or lower back, *stop.*

Equipment:

Pilates or yoga mat.

The Roll-Up

This movement stretches and strengthens the spine and abdominals and improves posture.

1. Lie on your back and extend your body into a full stretch with arms extended back over your head, legs together and straight. Squeeze your buttocks tightly and press the backs of the inner thighs together.

2. Inhale, drawing in the abdominals, and lift your straight arms toward the ceiling. Continue the movement forward.

3. As your arms pass over your chest, begin to roll up, bringing your chin toward your chest, lifting your head and the backs of your shoulders off the mat. Concentrate on drawing in your abdominals. Use the resistance of the floor and roll up your spine, articulating each spinal segment, vertebra by vertebra, while

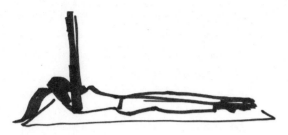

maintaining the C-curve of the spine and still-ness in your lower body.

Remember: Do not roll up using your neck or shoulders. Draw the weight of your head forward with your chin tucked as you articulate forward and back through the spine. The head follows the natural curve of the spine. You may place your neck at risk if you leave your head behind you when curling up. The movement should appear effortless and the curve of the body consistent.

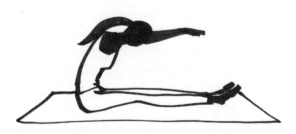

4. Exhale; continue curling your chest over your ribs, ribs over your hips. Try to lift up out of your hips and over your thighs as you pass through a sitting position. Exhale as you stretch forward, keeping your navel pulled back into your spine with your fingers reaching toward your toes.

5. Inhale; begin to roll back down until your lower back connects with the mat. Again, squeeze

your buttocks and inner thighs for stabilization as you roll through the spine with a slight tuck of your tailbone under, abs engaged. When your upper back touches the mat, lower your head and extend your arms to the starting position before beginning again.

Repeat 3 to 5 times. Perform the move slowly in a controlled way, engaging the muscles of your powerhouse throughout.

Modification

If you are unable to come to a sitting position with good form, follow the modified instruction as follows:

1. Lie on your back with your feet firmly on the floor and knees bent. Place your hands behind the backs of your thighs for support while rolling up to help lift your upper trunk. Maintain the C-curve when lifting off the mat and in the sitting position.

2. In the top (sitting) position with your shoulders directly over your hips, maintain the C-curve, extending your arms and legs to straight. Complete the stretch forward as far as you can go comfortably with good form as you exhale, stretching the muscles of your back and legs.

3. When rolling back down, bend your knees again and place your hands behind your thighs for support.

4. You can also shorten the range of motion by stopping when you're sitting upright.

The Hundred

This abdominal and breathing exercise is meant to circulate the blood and warm up the body. The Hundred is one of the Pilates method's signature abdominal exercises that highlight the powerhouse.

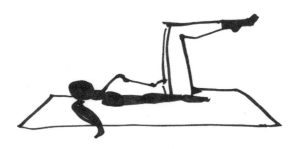

1. Start by lying on your back with your knees and hips bent at 90 degrees (tabletop position) and your arms resting on the mat beside you.

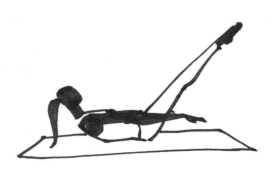

2. Exhale, draw your abdominals in, and lift your upper spine, reaching your arms forward, slightly above the mat. Straighten and extend your legs to a 45- to 60-degree angle, or the appropriate height for you, by keeping your legs at a height that gives you the abdominal strength and control to support the extension and keep your spine connected with the mat. The higher your legs, the less challenging. Keep in mind that muscle strength and control increase with practice. You can start with your feet on the floor or your legs in the table-top position, decreasing the demand on your abdominals. You can lower your legs closer to the floor as your practice develops. Focus on maintaining a firm abdominal contraction so your lower back remains pressed into the mat.

3. Begin pumping your arms straight down then up on each count for a total of 5 counts, inhaling for the duration of 5 and exhaling for 5, reaching forward as you breathe. Make sure you pump your entire arms and not just the hands breaking at the wrists.

4. Maintain this position, pumping your arms and breathing for 100 counts as long as good form can be maintained. Squeezing your buttocks and the backs of your inner thighs together will provide stability. Keep your shoulders pressed down away from your ears.

Remember: If your neck hurts, lower your head and neck to the mat and then try again. Make sure you are not lifting from the neck itself.

Modification

If you are finding core stability difficult—that is, if it's a challenge for you to maintain a constant position of spinal flexion (drawing in your abdominal muscles during the exercise and imprinting your lower back into the mat) when your legs are off the floor and neck and shoulders relaxed—then try the modifications that follow and slowly progress to a more challenging leg position.

Extend your legs straight to the ceiling rather than holding them at a 45- or 60-degree angle; or you can bend your knees and place your feet flat on the mat.

Variation

Add a small exercise or playground ball between your thighs and squeeze while performing the exercise.

Single Leg Stretch

This is a valuable stability exercise emphasizing the abdominals. Core stability means being able to maintain the appropriate positioning and activation of the core during movement. In other words, you can keep your pelvis and spine in the desired position while moving your limbs or whole body without compensating via changing form. The powerhouse serves as the engine that drives the movement. The leg movement is independent of the pelvis.

Lie on your back with your head and shoulders off the mat, chin toward your chest and right knee pulled into your chest with your inside hand (left) on your knee and your outside hand (right) on your ankle, elbows extended. The straight leg is extended in front of you at a height that allows your back to remain flat on the mat.

Inhale as you begin to bend your straight leg and straighten your bent leg.

Exhale as you complete the switch. Your hands switch to the opposite knee and ankle. Remember to stay lifted and forward in your upper trunk. Maintain core stability while executing, with your abdominals drawn in and your spine pressed into the mat. Repeat the sequence 5 times on each leg for a total of 10 times.

Remember: Keep the shoulders pressed down away from your ears. It's important that the position of the head be aligned with the spine.

Modification

You can perform this exercise with your bent leg just beyond vertical rather than into the chest. If you have a bad back, extend your straight leg to the ceiling.

Variation

Perform the Single Leg Stretch while keeping both legs straight. This adds the benefits of a dynamic hamstring stretch and a deepening of the abdominal contraction.

1. Inhaling, start by lying on your back, with your head and the backs of your shoulders rolled off the mat toward your chest. Straighten both legs to the ceiling.

2. As you continue inhaling, place your hands behind your right calf (or ankle if you can reach). Lower your left leg toward the mat to a height that allows you to keep your back flat on the mat. If this is too challenging, lower your leg onto the mat.

3. Exhaling, draw your right leg slightly closer to your face, deepening the abdominal contraction. Pulse your leg twice.

4. Inhaling, switch your straight legs simultaneously. Lower your right leg to the mat and your left toward your face. The switch should be quick; maintain absolute stillness in your torso. Continue alternating legs.

Repeat the sequence 5 times on each leg for a total of 20 reps. Lowering a straight leg requires a strong abdominal contraction.

Remember: This exercise offers many options to accommodate individual needs. If the stretch in the hamstrings is difficult in the beginning, you can hold your legs lower down—at the backs of your thighs, but not behind the knees. If you have weaker abdominal muscles, you can switch legs one at a time. As you gain strength, perform the switch with both legs simultaneously.

Crisscross

This exercise works the obliques, the waistline, and the powerhouse.

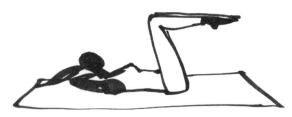

1. Lie on your back with your head and shoulders lifted off the mat, knees bent into your chest and hands behind your head, elbows wide.

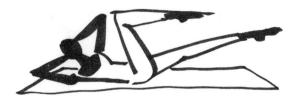

2. Exhale. Straighten one leg while simultaneously rotating your upper body toward the opposite bent knee.

3. Inhale as you begin to switch legs while your upper torso rotates back to center.

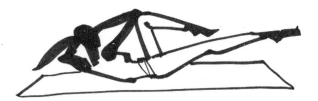

4. While switching legs, rotate your trunk toward the opposite side and exhale as you fully straighten one leg and bend the other toward your chest. Stay lifted when you rotate. Complete 5 to 10 sets.

Remember: Pull your navel to your spine and maintain the connection of your lower back and pelvis with the mat throughout the exercise. Do not rock from hip to hip in the direction of the rotation.

Make sure you are lifting and twisting from your waist, not from your neck and shoulders. The rotation of the trunk is key, because it emphasizes the work of the obliques.

Keep your elbows extended and look back at your elbows as you rotate.

Leg Pull

The leg pull strengthens the abs, arms, legs, and buttocks.

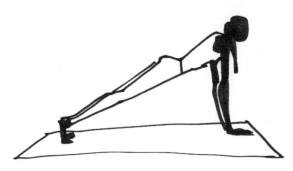

1. Start in the push-up position with your body weight supported on your hands and toes (curled under) and your heels pressed back. Your hands should be directly under your shoulders. You can also start on your knees and extend one leg out at a time into position.

Focus on pressing your arms into the mat, pushing away from the heels of your hands so that you do not sink into your wrists.

2. Squeeze your buttocks and concentrate on using your abdominals to stabilize your lower body. Your body should be in one straight line from the top of the head to your heels.

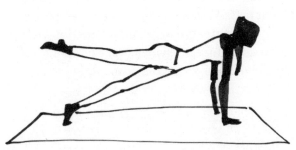

Be conscious not to sink into your back. Press your shoulders down away from your ears.

3. Inhaling, raise one leg toward the ceiling, squeezing the buttocks. Do not lift your hip when lifting your leg.

4. Exhaling, lower your leg back to the mat.

5. Inhaling, raise the opposite leg.

6. Exhaling, lower that leg back down.

Remember: Keep your abdominals engaged and pelvis lifted to prevent your lower back from arching.

Modifications

Modify the plank position by lowering your forearms onto the mat with your elbows directly beneath your shoulders.

Or lower onto your knees instead of balancing on your toes.

You can also just hold the plank without the leg extensions.

Variation

Lift and extend your right leg off the mat, squeeze your buttocks at the top of the extension (maintaining constant engagement), and pulse the leg 5 times. Switch legs and repeat. Perform the movements with precision.

BUILD-A-WORKOUT

Gunnar Peterson is a world-renowned personal trainer based in Beverly Hills who has worked with celebrities, athletes from the NBA, NHL, NFL, and USTA, and everyday people for more than twenty years. I asked him to design a program to help you incorporate strength training into your life, and he has come up with an ingenious one that will help you ease into exercise if you need to take it slow. Just as you add treatments to your at-home skin care regimen, you will add exercises and increase sets and repetitions as you progress from Solo, Couple, Triplet, and Quartet to Quintuplet. Trust yourself to the expertise of a phenomenal trainer:

Start with 2 sets of the movement(s) you choose and do 10 to 20 reps depending on your level. Work up to 3 to 4 sets of 15 to 20 perfect reps two to four times per week.

It's better to do fewer reps in perfect form than to rush through sloppy reps. If you are a total novice and do 2 sets of the five moves, it will take you twelve to fifteen minutes. If you do 4 sets of the five exercises, it should take twenty to thirty minutes depending on how proficient you become before tacking on sets. You are going to need to prioritize this workout if you want to reap the rewards.

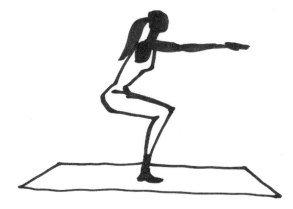

Solo: Squats

The squat involves lowering yourself toward the floor without bending at the lower back. Instead, you use your legs to lower your body, keeping your spine in a neutral position.

1. Stand with your feet hip-width apart.

2. Press your hips back and bend your knees. Keep your weight back on your heels, not on the balls of your feet. Your knees should stay behind your toes. Continue lowering until your knees are at almost a 90-degree bend.

3. Pause for a beat and then push through your heels, extending your knees and hips. The National Strength and Conditioning Association calls this the "King of all exercises." You just took their king; congratulations!

Couple: Squats, Then Push-Ups

Squats (see above).

Push-Ups

1. Place your hands on the floor so that they are slightly outside shoulder-width. Spread your fingers slightly out and have them pointed forward.

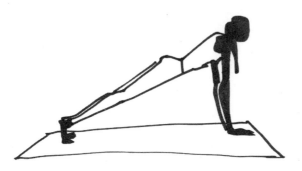

2. Rise up onto your toes so that all of your body weight is on your hands and your feet. Contract your abdominals to keep your torso in a straight line and to prevent arching your back or pointing your bottom in the air.

Variations: You can put your hands on the back of the sofa if you need to work your way up to the Full Monty! Another easier variation on the push-up is to start on your knees with the rest of the form remaining the same. Whichever works for you works for me, as long as you are working!

3. Bend your elbows and lower your chest toward the floor.

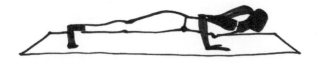

4. Once your elbows bend to 90 degrees, push off through your hands and extend your arms so that you return to the starting position. Push off as if you were getting off a hot surface! Effort is what wins the day!

Triplet: Squats, Push-Ups, Crunches

Squats, push-ups (see above).

Crunches

1. Lie on a flat surface with your lower back curvature pressed against the surface. Your feet should be bent at the knee and pressed firmly against the floor. Your arms should be either kept alongside your body or crossed on top of your chest—these positions avoid neck strain.

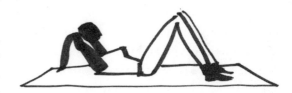

2. With your hips stationary, flex your waist by contracting your abdominals; curl your shoulders and trunk upward until you feel a nice contraction in your abdominals. Your arms should simply slide up the sides of your legs (if you have them at your sides) or stay on top of your chest (if you have them crossed). Your lower back should always remain in contact with the floor. Exhale as you perform this movement and hold the contraction for a second.

3. As you inhale, go back to the starting position.

The strengthening of your core musculature will aid in pain relief—and the aesthetic benefits aren't too shabby, either.

Quartet: Squats, Push-Ups, Crunches, Lateral Hops to One Leg

Squats, push-ups, crunches (see above).

Lateral Hops to One Leg

1. Stand on one leg with a slight bend in your knee. Your other foot is *not* in contact with the floor.

2. Now switch feet.

3. Next, add a little spring to your step as you hop to the other foot.

As you become more competent and confident in this move, make it more explosive in the takeoff and sink slightly as you absorb the landing to make those strong leg muscles contract eccentrically. Now you're getting there!

Quintuplet: Squats, Push-Ups, Crunches, Lateral Hops, Plank

Squats, push-ups, crunches, lateral hops (see above).

Plank

1. Lie facedown on the mat, resting on your forearms, palms flat on the floor.

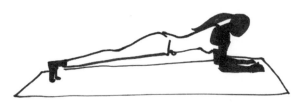

2. Push off the floor, raising up onto your toes and resting on your elbows. Keep your back flat, in a straight line from head to heels. Tilt your pelvis and contract your abdominals to prevent your rear end from sticking up in the air or sagging in the middle.

3. Hold for 5, 10, or on up to 60 seconds, depending on your level.

Your posture will benefit hugely from this move. And carrying yourself upright speaks of confidence, which has a huge ripple effect on your life!

Add fifteen to forty-five minutes of walking to any of these levels. Do what you can on a given day, but be honest. If you have only fifteen minutes, use them, but if you actually have forty-five minutes, do that! Don't cheat yourself!

If you follow my recommendations for the Lancer Anti-Aging Lifestyle—managing stress, eating whole, fresh foods and avoiding those that age you, and becoming more physically active—you will be transformed. You will establish a new source of energy to tap that will make you clear and light. Your radiance will shine from the inside. Combining an anti-aging lifestyle with the appropriate Lancer Skincare regimen will take you to a place of confidence, exhilaration, and ageless beauty. You will be in top form. Your appeal will be dazzling. As I said at the very start of *Younger: The Breakthrough Anti-Aging Method for Radiant Skin*, attraction is the driving force within us all.

Afterword

Now that you have read *Younger*, I consider you an associate patient of Lancer Dermatology. As I am sure you have noticed, our involvement with our patients goes well beyond consultations and treatments in the office. We give our patients the cell phone numbers of key staff members to contact in case they have questions regarding skin care products or procedures. We monitor the progress of everyone who comes to the office and answer questions from those who use our products. Patients send photographs of changing conditions from their phones. We have to respond to changes. Follow-up is important.

I want you to have similar access to the experts at Lancer Dermatology. I hope you will send any questions you might have to my website: www.lancerskincare .com. We will do our best to answer you and give you guidance if you need it. We always welcome personal stories and want to know what has worked for you. Of course, we are excited by descriptions of transformations. It will be gratifying to know my work is helping others beyond my practice in Beverly Hills. Follow me on Twitter or Facebook.

Lancer Skincare is located at:
440 Rodeo Drive
Beverly Hills, CA 90210
800-899-0744

If reading this book keeps you from acting impulsively and regretting it by educating you about the pitfalls of the anti-aging beauty trap, I have accomplished what I intended. Rather than buying into the fantasy of eternal youth, you should have more realistic expectations. You understand that looking younger begins at home with the Lancer Skincare regimen that is right for your skin. Knowing about the biology of aging should inspire you to adopt a healthier lifestyle, because all the skin care products and procedures in the world will not be effective if you do not fight aging from within. Once you prepare the canvas through skin care, you might want to continue your anti-aging campaign by trying some non-invasive procedures to improve your skin even more. Most of my patients do, even those who are initially reluctant. They are so thrilled by how great they look with just skin care and lifestyle changes that they decide to take it as far as they can with in-office procedures. They notice that the world is responding differently to them, and they like it. As their confidence grows, they want to boost their appeal even more. They are not making decisions out of insecurity or flaw obsession. They are proceeding in the most positive way, feeling good about themselves and what they have already accomplished. As I said at the start of the book, everyone wants to look younger, because nothing is more attractive than vitality and radiance.

By now, you should be persuaded that only a board-certified dermatologist is qualified to plan and execute a personalized, step-by-step program to prevent and reverse signs of aging for you. Forget what your friends are doing or the latest quick fix in this month's fashion magazine. Find a conservative dermatologist to guide you, one who is not pushing procedures and is prepared to take baby steps to get you where you want to be. Do not get talked into procedures you do not want. If you are not happy with your consultation, try another dermatologist. You will be collaborating with this physician for long-term restoration and rejuvenation. Trust and follow-through are essential. Go with your instincts and what you have learned in *Younger*, and you will not go wrong.

Appendixes

Beyond Home Care

For twelve chapters, you have been reading about my approach to looking younger. Restoration and rejuvenation instead of renovation are the way to go. I am glad to say that a shift is happening in the world of cosmetic procedures. Advances in technology have made minimally invasive procedures more and more effective. They are less expensive, they require significantly less time for recuperation, and the risk of complications from the procedures is much lower than from surgery. Even so, the procedures are only as good as the professional performing them. That is why it's so important to find a board-certified dermatologist to guide you on a path that is right for you.

Everyone wants to get in on the action in this lucrative field, because the demand is so high. From aestheticians and nurses at medi-spas to physicians who have not specialized in dermatology, unqualified people everywhere will be selling you hard on neurotoxins, fillers, and laser resurfacing with the promise of firming, toning, and lifting the skin. Do not allow yourself to become a victim. One size definitely does not fit all when it comes to anti-aging. You need to have an experienced and careful dermatologist guide you through the morass of products and treatments, tailoring an individualized program for you.

In planning the most effective way to treat patients, I have to use the six dimensions of aging to determine the best treatment approach for each individual. I have to take into account what a patient wants to achieve, what is motivating the patient to change, what the patient expects from the treatment, and how much effort that patient is willing to put into an anti-aging program. It makes no sense to plan a multi-step regimen and a long-term treatment plan if there is no way a particular patient will be compliant.

When we work with patients, our approach is holistic. I cannot treat the skin without trying to pinpoint underlying causes for the skin problems and helping patients to resolve them. Lifestyle corrections are a big part of treatment plans. The stories that follow will show you how much can be accomplished through skin care and medical rehabilitation.

A BRIEF OVERVIEW OF PROCEDURES

After you have reaped the benefits of the Lancer Method program, you might be interested in taking the improvements a step further by supporting your good work with minimally invasive in-office procedures. These rejuvenating procedures range from chemical peels to laser resurfacing, from fillers to radio wave and ultrasound skin tightening. Your dermatologist will adjust the many, complex settings of the treatment equipment, determine the correct blend of chemicals for your chemical peel, perform laser work, and properly inject fillers and neurotoxins. The proper use of injectables is an art form. No one but your dermatologist should perform a procedure that penetrates your skin. Though they may be medically knowledgeable, nurses, physician's assistants, and aestheticians should not be giving you fillers or neurotoxins. In my office, I am the only one to do these procedures. In some instances, such as radio wave or ultrasound skin tightening, I set the equipment for the specific patient right before the procedure is to begin. A nurse may perform the treatment, but I do check in regularly to oversee the procedure. Do not accept anything less from your physician. Your doctor has to be directly involved every step of the way.

I will not be using brand names in the procedure descriptions, mainly because technological advances are happening at such a rapid pace, with equipment and procedures constantly being superseded by the "newest" advances. My office is inundated with salespeople and elaborate mailings exclaiming about the latest breakthrough techniques. Cosmetic surgery for anti-aging purposes is about to become obsolete, and this is progress worth applauding in my opinion. Here is a rundown of non-invasive treatments available right now.

Microdermabrasion

This is a quick and easy way to revitalize your skin in less than thirty minutes. It works for all LES types. A minimally abrasive instrument is used to sand the skin, removing the thick, uneven outer layer. The mild abrasion is followed by vacuum suction to remove the loosened dead skin cells. Microdermabrasion is used to treat sun damage, age spots, superficial pigmentation, fine lines, wrinkles, stretch marks, mild acne scars, blackheads, whiteheads, and clogged pores. The technique stimulates collagen production and leaves your skin looking fresh and vibrant. There is no downtime or recovery period, but your skin will be more sensitive to sun exposure after this procedure, so be sure to use sunscreen immediately following a microdermabrasion session.

Skin Tightening

Without damaging the skin's surface, pulsed light therapy (also known as phototherapy) heats the epidermis and dermis and stimulates the formation of collagen. Skin tightening is the result.

Radio frequency and ultrasound can also be used to firm, tighten, and lift the skin without injuring its surface. These therapies address the foundational layer of skin that lifts and supports the outer layers.

In each case, energy—from radio frequency, ultrasound, or light—heats the fibrous tissue in the dermis and subcutaneous levels. The heat breaks down collagen and elastin and causes these fibers to contract. This shrinking results in tightening, firming, and subtle lifting. The body's natural wound-healing response kicks in, and more collagen is produced.

No time is needed to recuperate from skin tightening treatments, which are usually performed in a series for optimal results. Your skin will continue to tighten for up to six months after the treatments as the collagen-building process continues. The ultimate lifting and toning occur during the three-month period following the treatment as new collagen is created. Ultrasound therapy has the additional benefit of allowing the physician to see the layers of tissue being targeted during treatment.

Laser Resurfacing

Ablative laser therapy is used to remove top layers of the epidermis to produce smoother, fresher skin. The laser triggers new cell growth and damage repair. Non-ablative laser treatments that are more precisely targeted are used more frequently today.

Laser therapy now uses concentrated, pulsating beams of light aimed at irregularities in the skin. The process removes unwanted, damaged skin in a very precise manner one layer at a time. People with LES IV or more should be very cautious about having laser treatments, as they can cause permanent discoloration.

Laser Fractionated Restoration is a treatment we use at Lancer Skincare. With this new therapy, only a fraction of the skin receives the laser light. The laser directs closely spaced, microscopic beams to the trouble spots while preserving normal healthy skin between the laser spots. The preservation of healthy skin results in rapid healing. Laser resurfacing can improve fine lines and wrinkles around the eyes, forehead, and mouth, sun damage, age spots, acne or chickenpox scars, and enlarged oil glands on the nose.

CO_2 laser resurfacing delivers very short pulsed light energy or continuous light beams. This type of laser removes thin layers of skin with little damage to surrounding tissue.

Erbium laser resurfacing is used to remove superficial and moderately deep lines and wrinkles on the face, but can also be used on the neck, chest, or hands.

Lasers are also used for hair and tattoo removal and for treating broken blood vessels.

Do not let anyone who is not an experienced physician do laser work on your skin. There are many different types of lasers. The machines have to be set for frequency, energy, fluence, power, penetration, beam configuration, depth of penetration, and diameter of the beam. You need a specialist who knows how to set up the equipment in the right way for your skin.

Chemical Peels

One of the least invasive ways to improve the appearance of your skin, chemical peeling, uses chemical solutions to improve and smooth its texture by removing damaged outer layers. Your doctor will use a formula that has been adjusted for your needs. The concentrations of the chemicals result in light, medium, or deep peels.

- Light peels improve uneven pigment, dryness, acne, or fine wrinkling. This level of peel offers a light exfoliation. The chemicals often used are alpha and beta hydroxy acids, glycolic acid, lactic acid, salicylic acid, and maleic acid, which are all mild. You will need up to six treatments for the full benefit of a light peel.
- Medium chemical peels are used for uneven skin tone, acne scars, and deeper wrinkles. This type of peel will remove skin cells from the epidermis and the upper part of the dermis. A combination of trichloroacetic acid and

glycolic acid is used. The skin of the treated area may turn red or brown after the peel and take up to six weeks to heal.

- Deep chemical peels have dramatic results. They are used for deep facial wrinkles, sun damage, scars, blotchiness, and pre-cancerous growths. Phenol is often used to penetrate to the lower dermal layers. You will need a local anesthetic and a sedative to manage discomfort. There is an eight-week pre-treatment period that may include the use of a prescription medication derived from vitamin A. After the chemicals are neutralized, the treated area is covered with a soothing gel. The area will be swollen and uncomfortable. The swelling will go down in two weeks, but your skin may be red for up to three months. The good news is that the benefits from one treatment can last for years.

Neurotoxins

The best-known neurotoxin, botulinum toxin, more commonly known by its brand name, Botox, has changed the way the world looks at cosmetic procedures. More than 3.3 million treatments with botulinum toxin were done in the United States in 2012. This substance is the most popular way to reduce facial wrinkles, smoothing crow's-feet, frown lines, forehead furrows, and skin bands on the neck. The neurotoxins used are derived from bacteria that have been purified. When injected, the neurotoxin blocks muscular nerve signals, which weakens the muscle so that it cannot contract and thus diminishes unwanted wrinkles.

Using neurotoxins well is an art and a science. There are forty-three muscles in your face. The person giving you the injections has to understand and pinpoint the correct spots to optimize your treatment. For example, for jawline firming, I often inject small amounts of Botox on either side of the jaw, which might seem counterintuitive. When the jaw muscles relax, the cheek muscles pull up in a rubber band action, which lifts the sag along the jaw. You need an artist and an architect to sculpt and balance the supports of your face to fight aging. Otherwise, you might end up looking as if you have come out of deep freeze with a face that does not move.

Fillers

Large-volume fillers are the latest in facial rejuvenation, but I am not talking about goldfish lips. New technology and a better understanding of the aging face have advanced the use of fillers to restore the shape of the face. Sunken cheeks, jowls, and protruding bones add years to your face. I always say that after age twenty-five, facial fat diminishes. Fillers can restore the volume that decreases with age. There are many fillers on the market, some suitable for treating fine lines and wrinkles and others more appropriate for a larger correction. Here are some of the popular large-volume fillers:

Fat transfer takes fat from one area of your body, processes it, and redeposits it in the desired location. You are using your own natural fat and stem cells, so your body will not reject the filler substance. This procedure may have unpredictable results and can be lumpier than desired.

Collagen fillers were the first type of dermal fillers on the market to be used in aesthetic procedures, particularly for lip injections. Collagen fillers are derived from human skin or animals, namely, cows and pigs. Patient self-derived collagen is available, but this process of collagen transfer is infrequently used.

Hyaluronic acid is found throughout the body. Attracting water, this acid hydrates and plumps the skin. These popular fillers are used in a thin version for fine lines and lip augmentation. Thicker versions are used for more extensive procedures. When this gel is injected, it acts like an inflated cushion to support facial structures and tissues that may have lost elasticity or volume. Hyaluronic acid brings water to the skin's surface, keeping it supple and fresh-looking.

Calcium hydroxyapatite spheres suspended in a gel stimulate the growth of collagen and improve the skin immediately upon their injection. This filler, the heaviest of dermal fillers, is a good choice for deep lines. Calcium hydroxyapatite contains small particles that act as a scaffold. Your own collagen grows on that scaffold, and eventually the particles dissolve.

Polylactic acid is used extensively for facial volume replacement. The product is administered in a series of injections over several months and works deep in the dermis to replace lost collagen. The effect can last two years.

Polyalkylimide is a synthetic material often used for such deep wrinkles as nasolabial folds or depressed scars and to enhance cheekbones and the jawline. It is not used for fine wrinkles. You receive a local anesthetic, and the material is injected under your skin and molded into place. A thin layer of collagen slowly forms around it over the course of about a month. A large volume can be used, and it is stable. It can also be removed if necessary.

PMMA is used to treat medium to deep wrinkles, folds, and furrows, to augment thin lips, and to fill out pitted scars. The PMMA microspheres are suspended in a solution of purified collagen gel. PMMA is the longest-lasting filler. A number of injections are needed to create volume, taking up to three months to reach full effect. PMMA can sometimes be visible under the skin. This product is also difficult to remove.

Once again, you need a highly skilled doctor to inject your face with fillers. You cannot imagine some of the disasters I have been asked to fix. Some people come to my office looking like a Picasso painting for all the wrong reasons. The risks include:

- Acne
- Rejection of filler material
- Under- or overcorrection of wrinkles
- Bruising
- Asymmetry
- Itching
- Infection at injection site
- Redness
- Rashes
- Sensitivity
- Swelling
- Temporary numbness
- Temporary paralysis of facial muscles
- Migration of filler material
- Clumping that results from facial movement or natural aging
- Anatomic distortion

In my opinion, fillers should not be permanent. The way your body absorbs the fillers and how your face continues to age will determine how often you need to repeat treatments.

Dermabrasion

This procedure is a more invasive form of refinishing the skin's top layers through controlled surgical scraping. A physician uses a wire brush or a diamond wheel with rough edges to remove the upper layers of skin. A local anesthetic is used for the procedures. The process injures the skin, causing it to bleed and stimulating the healing process. The treatment softens the sharp edges of surface irregularities, making the skin appear smoother. Dark complexions—from LES IV to V—may become permanently discolored or blotchy after this treatment, so it is not right for everyone. If you have sensitive skin, you could experience flares. Dermabrasion is used to reduce scars, including deep acne scars, remove pre-cancerous growths, and smooth out fine facial wrinkles, such as those around the mouth. It is essential that an experienced board-certified physician perform this treatment.

Recovery and healing time depends on the size and depth of the treated area. In general, the regrowth of skin takes from five to eight days. The new skin will be pink or reddish and takes about six to twelve weeks to fade.

Your dermatologist might suggest using a combination of treatments to rejuvenate your skin. Remember to start slow and build up from the least invasive treatments to more intense procedures.

Appendix 2

The Lancer Skincare Products

I am proud of the Lancer Skincare products. A lot of thought and research have gone into the formulation of every product in the line. Lancer Skincare products are the ultimate in skin care, designed to address the root cause of aging skin: the gradual slowing down of the skin's ability to regenerate itself. The combination of the Lancer Method with Lancer Skincare products is unbeatable. The products have been created with interlocking chemistry. One product supports and boosts the effects of the others. The results are visible and dramatic. Skin that acts younger begins to look younger.

For a full description of these products, their ingredients, and what they are formulated to do, check our website, www.lancerskincare.com. You can find all the Lancer Skincare products at Bergdorf Goodman, Harrods, and select Nordstrom locations.

Microcurrent Power Boost

The Basic Lancer Method
The Method: Polish
The Method: Cleanse
The Method: Nourish

The Lancer Method for Blemish Control
The Method: Polish Blemish Control
The Method: Cleanse Blemish Control
The Method: Nourish Blemish Control

The Lancer Method for Sensitive Skin
The Method: Polish Sensitive Skin
The Method: Cleanse Sensitive Skin
The Method: Nourish Sensitive Skin

Lancer Skincare Advanced Treatments
Fade Serum Intense
Lift Serum Intense
Intensive Night Treatment
Eye Contour Lifting Cream
Sheer Fluid Sun Shield SPF 30
Retexturizing Treatment Cream
Advanced C Radiance Cream

Lancer Skincare Products Coming for Spring 2014
Regeneration Serum
The Method: Body Polish
The Method: Body Cleanse
The Method: Body Nourish

Index

About the Author

HAROLD A. LANCER, MD, FAAD, is the expert whom Hollywood's most recognizable faces trust to preserve and enhance their looks. In the past twenty-five years, Dr. Lancer's Beverly Hills practice has become a trusted brand for effective cosmetic rejuvenation.

Dr. Lancer is a medical graduate of the University of California–San Diego and completed his dermatology residency at Harvard Medical School. He later completed a plastic surgery fellowship at the Tel HaShomer Hospital in Tel Aviv, followed by clinics in London at St John's Hospital for Diseases of the Skin. He returned to Southern California and received his board certification in dermatology in 1983; there he started his solo practice. His clients fly from all over the world to receive his unique, cutting-edge treatments.

Published in many medical journals during the past thirty years, Dr. Lancer has served on the medical supervisory boards of Tridon Corporation, Epicuren, ORLY International, Edgar Morris Skin Care, Natren Inc., and Chanel Corporation. He also has affiliations with Cedars-Sinai Medical Center and UCLA Medical Center.